AF597957

Atlas of Pediatric Cardiac CTA

Randy Ray Richardson

Atlas of Pediatric Cardiac CTA

Congenital Heart Disease

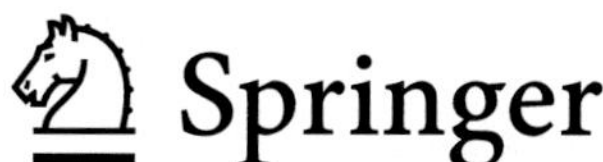

Springer

Randy Ray Richardson, MD
Department of Radiology
St. Joseph's Hospital and Medical Center
Creighton University School of Medicine
Phoenix, AZ, USA

ISBN 978-1-4614-0087-5 ISBN 978-1-4614-0088-2 (eBook)
DOI 10.1007/978-1-4614-0088-2
Springer New York Heidelberg Dordrecht London

Library of Congress Control Number: 2013938368

Printed on acid-free paper

Springer is part of Springer Science+Business Media (www.springer.com)

I would like to dedicate this book to my nephew, Mark Wright. Mark was born with hypoplastic left heart syndrome. He has spent months in the hospital with caring physicians and medical personnel who have helped him through multiple surgeries and procedures to develop a new physiology for his cardiovascular system. Fortunately for Mark, he has tolerated these surgeries and procedures well and is an active 4-year-old boy. It would be hard for anyone who didn't know his history to suspect he had any problems at all. As a radiologist, I rarely become emotionally involved in the lives of the patients I image. Mark helped me understand the myriad of emotions and stresses that a patient and his or her family go through as their child is treated for a serious congenital heart disease. Mark also helped me see the dedication of nurses and physicians who are so willing to give of their time and expertise, for which they never receive any monetary reimbursement. I am thankful for Mark, his family, and all those who participated in his care for teaching me these important lessons.

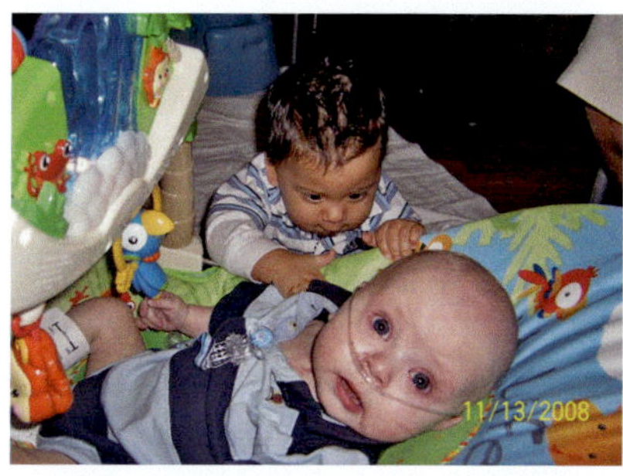

Fig. 1 Mark Wright (nephew) with oxygen tubing after his Glenn procedure, with cousin Riggs (behind)

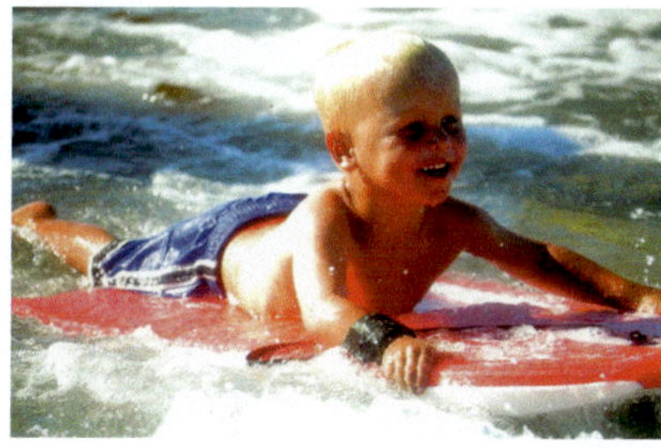

Fig. 2 Mark Wright at the beach after his third major open heart surgery

Preface

Atlas of Pediatric Cardiac CTA is a concise visual guide to the imaging of congenital heart disease in infants and children. Using an organized, systematic approach accompanied with clinical examples, the book focuses on the utilization of cardiac CTA imaging for pediatric patients distinct from adult patients, with an emphasis on techniques for prospective versus retrospective gated imaging, radiation lowering, adaptive statistical iterative reconstruction (ASIR), and modulation. The post-processing of cardiac CT information is also discussed, a method that results in maximizing the amount of information provided to the clinician. The final section of the book presents a systematic cardiac CTA evaluation search pattern, a useful guide for clinicians in assessing cardiac CTAs in infants and newborns. Since pediatric patients often present with multiple findings and complex anatomy, this discussion is broken down among the major structures of the cardiovascular system, with extensive imaging examples of situs anomalies, common lung and airway abnormalities, and findings involving the atria, ventricles, outflow tracts, great vessels, and coronary arteries. *The Atlas of Pediatric Cardiac CTA* is a valuable resource for radiologists, cardiologists, and other clinicians involved in the care of pediatric patients with congenital heart disease.

The following people have contributed to the details and understanding of these cases over the past several years during weekly conferences and individual discussions: Ernerio Alboliras, MD; Steve Pophal, MD; John Nigro, MD; David Cleveland, MD; Karim Diab, MD; Ed Rhee, MD; Lourdes Guerrero, MD; David Frakes, PhD; Fariha Ejaz; and Olga Kalinkin MD; Robert Puntel, MD; Christopher Derby, MD; Shabib Alhadheri, MD; Jeane Zenge, MD; Lawrence Lilien MD.

Phoenix, AZ Randy Ray Richardson, MD

Contents

Contributors

Ernerio T. Alboliras, MD Children's Heart Center, Phoenix Children's Hospital, Phoenix, AZ, USA

Todd Chapman, MD Radiology Residency Program, St. Joseph's Hospital and Medical Center, Phoenix, AZ, USA

Cam Chau, MD Radiology Residency Program, St. Joseph's Hospital and Medical Center, Phoenix, AZ, USA

Andrew Duarte, MD Radiology Residency Program, St. Joseph's Hospital and Medical Center, Phoenix, AZ, USA

Nhi Huynh, MD Radiology Residency Program, St. Joseph's Hospital and Medical Center, Phoenix, AZ, USA

Taruna Ralhan, MD Radiology Residency Program, St. Joseph's Hospital and Medical Center, Phoenix, AZ, USA

Randy Ray Richardson, MD Department of Radiology, St. Joseph's Hospital and Medical Center, Creighton University School of Medicine, Phoenix, AZ, USA

Travis Scharnweber, MD Radiology Residency Program, St. Joseph's Hospital and Medical Center, Phoenix, AZ, USA

1 Advantages of Cardiac CTA over Other Imaging Modalities

Randy Ray Richardson and Ernerio T. Alboliras

Congenital heart imaging has changed dramatically over the past several decades. In previous decades, plain x-ray films were a key diagnostic test, with the use of angiocardiography to make specific preoperative diagnoses. However, with several robust cross-sectional imaging modalities now available, this method no longer is the standard. Although plain films still are often obtained, they serve as more of a screening tool, with the first line of imaging being echocardiography. Echocardiography typically does not require sedation and does not expose the patient to ionizing radiation. Echocardiography provides detailed intracardiac anatomy with real-time functional evaluation; however, it may be limited for evaluating extracardiac structure. Similarly, cardiac MRI does not expose the patient to ionizing radiation and offers some of the best tools for functional evaluation of the heart. Cardiac CT angiography (CTA) is another cross-sectional imaging modality that may be used for anatomic and functional evaluation in patients with congenital heart disease. Cardiac CTA does require ionizing radiation; however, with new techniques designed to minimize the patient's exposure, the radiation can be kept within safe parameters and the advantages of CT may be used.

The advantages of cardiac CTA include the following:

1. Cardiac CTA produces the highest spatial resolution images of all three cross-sectional imaging modalities, which is an advantage for the following reasons:
   (a) In infants, CTA offers the best chance to visualize the coronary arteries, aortopulmonary collaterals, and pulmonary arteries. These vessels may be as small as 1–2 mm in diameter.
   (b) High–spatial resolution images allow the best postprocessing of anatomic detail for three-dimensional reconstructions, which often is important in patients with complex congenital heart disease, in whom anatomic relationships help in presurgical planning.
   (c) CTA gives the most accurate volumetric analysis of the ventricles, which may help determine the viability of a two-ventricle repair in a patient with a hypoplastic ventricle.
2. It is the modality of choice for evaluating coronary artery anomalies in infants.
   (a) Coronary artery anomalies are associated with congenital heart disease and may be important for presurgical planning. Even with the very rapid heart rate of an infant, a cardiac CT scan can reliably demonstrate the coronary arteries.

R.R. Richardson, MD (✉)
Department of Radiology,
St. Joseph's Hospital and Medical Center,
Creighton University School of Medicine,
West Thomas Rd 350, 85013 Phoenix, AZ, USA
e-mail: randy.richardson2@chw.edu,
randy.richardson2@dignityhealth.org

E.T. Alboliras, MD
Children's Heart Center,
Phoenix Children's Hospital,
Phoenix, AZ, USA

R.R. Richardson, *Atlas of Pediatric Cardiac CTA*,
DOI 10.1007/978-1-4614-0088-2_1, © Springer Science+Business Media New York 2013

   (b) Although other cross-sectional modalities often allow identification of the origins of the coronary arteries, cardiac CTA affords a more reliable evaluation of the course and termination of the coronary arteries.
3. It provides the best evaluation of the airway. Airway abnormalities frequently cause significant postoperative morbidity in congenital heart patients.
   (a) Congential airway anomalies are common in patients with congenital heart disease.
   (b) Airway compression from vascular anomalies, enlarged vessels (pulmonary arteries, patent ductus arteriosus, aorta), and cardiomegaly are common.
   (c) Bronchomalacia is a common finding in patients with congenital heart disease.
4. Cardiac CT requires short anesthesia times, and a typical scan takes seconds to perform. Short anesthesia times are an advantage in the complex congenital heart patient, in whom anesthesia management may be very difficult for long periods of time outside the intensive care unit. A typical cardiac CTA takes 4–5 s of scanning time. Anesthesia is needed to optimize the scan, with a breathhold required to stop all chest movement.

2 Scanning Technique for Cardiac CTA in Infants and Small Children

Randy Ray Richardson and Cam Chau

To fully utilize the advantages of cardiac CTA, it is important to consider radiation exposure and to optimize scanning techniques. Recent advances in multidetector CT (MDCT) technology have revolutionized cardiovascular imaging in children with complex congenital heart disease. For infants with congenital heart disease, ECG-gated cardiac CTA is the modality of choice for imaging the coronary arteries, airway, and extracardiac vascular structures. Fast scanning times and high-quality evaluation of both complex cardiac and coronary anatomy have enabled CTA to aid in patient management and treatment planning. Currently, there are two accepted cardiac CTA scanning techniques for infants with congenital heart disease: retrospective and prospective ECG-gated scanning.

Technique

General anesthesia is administered routinely in infants less than 1 year of age to optimize the scans. All examinations are performed with multidetector scanners. The following parameters are given for a GE 64-slice MDCT: 4 cm detector length. Iodinated contrast medium is used at 1 mL/lb of body weight, with an injection speed of 0.7 mL/s. A weight-based protocol is used, with 80-kVp tube voltage and tube current adjusted according to body weight for prospective scanning. Tube current adjustment to body weight varies from institution to institution and may range from 10 to 40 mA/kg [1, 2]. The gantry speed is set at a 0.35-s rotation with a helical thickness of 0.6 mm and detector coverage of 40 mm. The technologist begins the scan when contrast fills the ventricle. The patient is scanned in a craniocaudal direction starting at the level of the subclavian artery and ending at the level of the diaphragm. The anesthesiologist assists with the breath hold. β-Blockers typically are not used to decrease the heart rate in children with congenital heart disease.

Retrospective Scanning

During retrospective scanning, the x-ray beam is turned on during the entire cardiac cycle and spiral scanning continues during table motion (Fig. 2.1). Retrospective gating uses a low pitch (0.2) to obtain attenuation measurements at all spatial locations in the heart and to scan during all phases of the cardiac cycle, including the entire R-R interval. The pitch in retrospective scanning depends on the heart rate. Pitch normally falls in the range of 0.2–0.24 for infants with heart rates above 100 bpm. The current in retrospective scanning is set at 250–300 mA.

R.R. Richardson, MD (✉)
Department of Radiology, St. Joseph's Hospital and Medical Center, Creighton University School of Medicine, West Thomas Rd 350, 85013 Phoenix, AZ, USA
e-mail: randy.richardson2@chw.edu, randy.richardson2@dignityhealth.org

C. Chau, MD
Radiology Residency Program, St. Joseph's Hospital and Medical Center, Phoenix, AZ, USA

R.R. Richardson, *Atlas of Pediatric Cardiac CTA*,
DOI 10.1007/978-1-4614-0088-2_2, © Springer Science+Business Media New York 2013

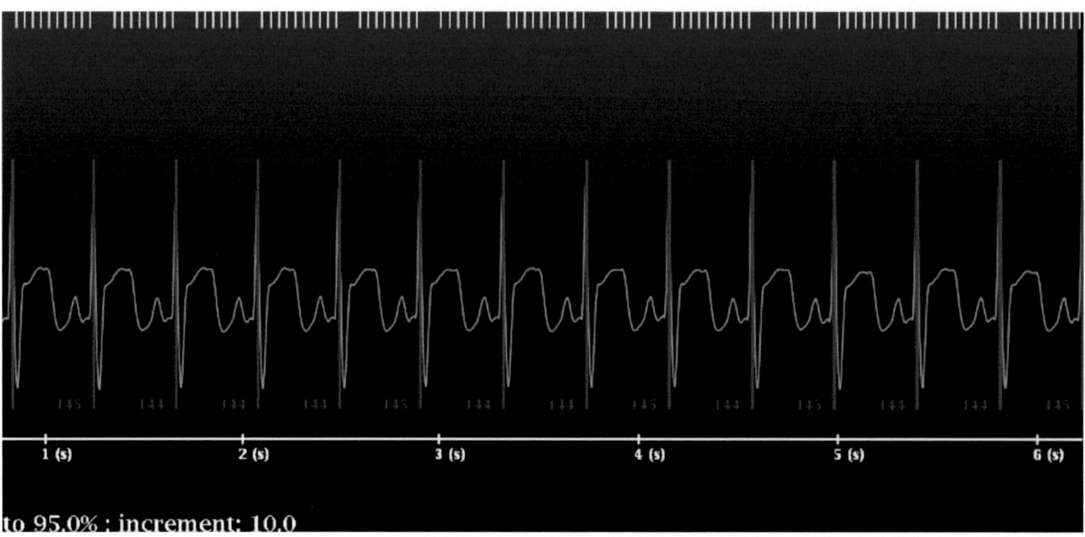

Fig. 2.1 Retrospective ECG-gated scan. The x-ray beam (in *blue*) is on through the entire cardiac cycle

Prospective Scanning

The vast majority of scanning can and should be done using the prospective ECG-triggered scanning technique, even in children and infants with very fast heart rates. This technique uses a nonspiral step-and-shoot axial scanning process in which the x-ray beam is on for a short time and is turned off as the table moves. The imaging window is approximately 50 % of the cardiac cycle. Because an infant's heart rate is relatively high, short acquisition times with padding may be used to capture up to 50 % of the cardiac cycle to evaluate function (Fig. 2.2); when functional analysis is needed, 175 ms of padding should be used. The padding turns the tube on before the required acquisition time and leaves it on afterward, increasing the time the current is on to include more of the cardiac cycle (Fig. 2.3) for functional imaging. For prospective scanning, our tube current–body weight adjustment has three weight based settings. Typically, end systole is the time for imaging the coronary arteries in adults, with optimal visualization between 65 and 80 % of the cardiac cycle. In infants, the optimal time for imaging the coronary arteries typically is during systole, at 45–55 % of the cardiac cycle.

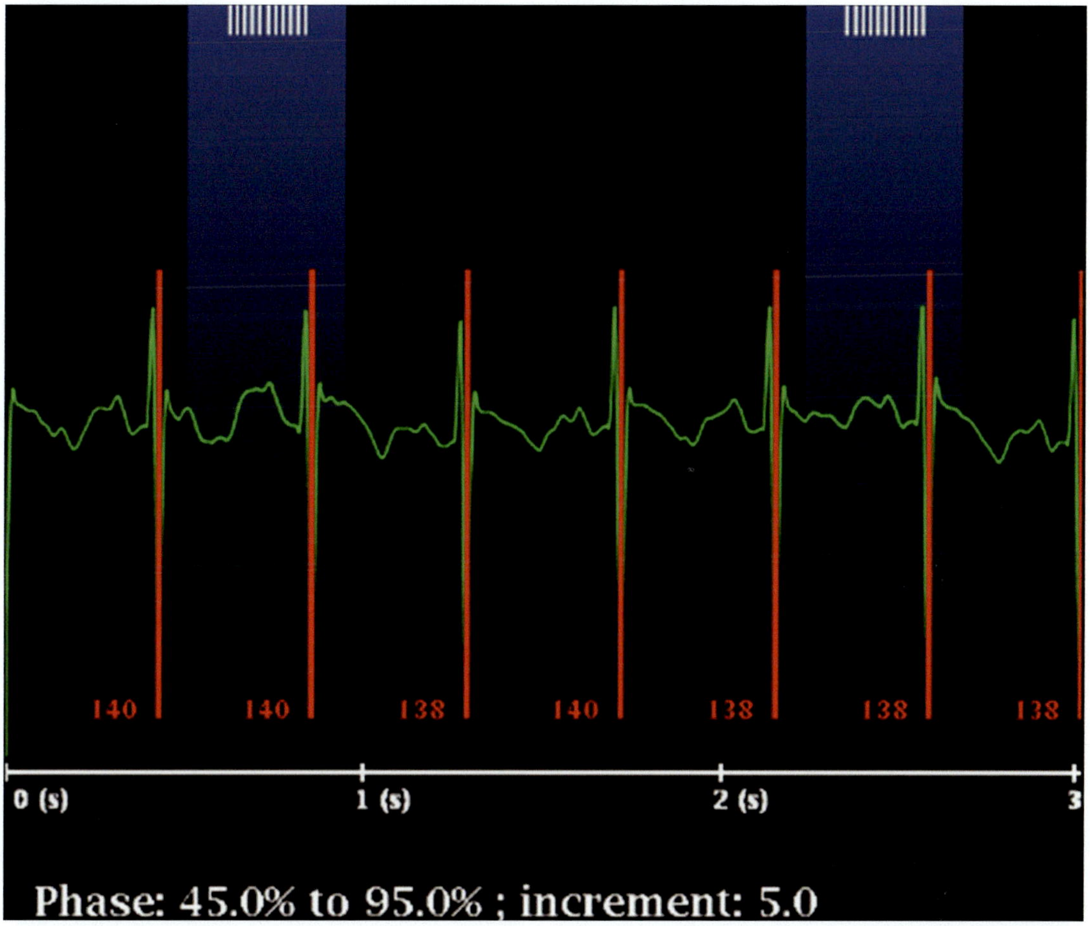

Fig. 2.2 Prospective ECG-gated scan. The x-ray beam (in *blue*) is not on during the entire cardiac cycle. Notice the rapid heart rate of 140 bpm. The rapid heart rate is advantage as the scan time covers enough of the cardiac cycle so that functional information can be obtained with provided with postprocessing

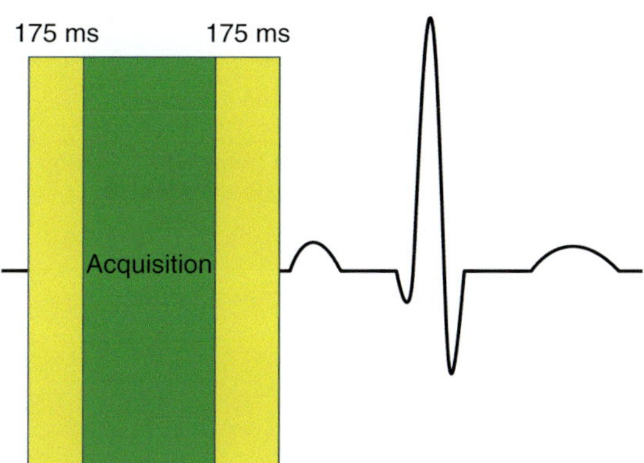

Fig. 2.3 Padding. Padding of 175 ms (*yellow*) is used to flank the acquisition time (*green*) to include more cardiac phases

Prospective Versus Retrospective Scanning (Table 2.1)

Table 2.1 Retrospective versus prospective ECG-gated scanning

Retrospective	Prospective
Scans the entire cardiac cycle	Scans a variable portion of the cardiac cycle based on the padding time
X-ray beam is *on* the entire time	X-ray beam is *not* on the entire time
No padding is used	Padding may be used to cover parts of the cardiac cycle to obtain functional information
Higher radiation dose	Lower radiation dose

Radiation Dose

Children are more sensitive than adults to the effects of ionizing radiation; therefore, it is essential to balance image quality with radiation dose delivered when performing CTA in children. It is important to apply the ALARA (As Low As Reasonably Achievable) principle for infants and neonates by using low peak kilovoltage and adapting the milliamperes to the patient's weight. Published studies comparing retrospective with prospective ECG-gated scanning techniques have reported radiation dose savings ranging from two to four times with prospective ECG-gated techniques [1–4]. Radiation doses estimated for prospective ECG-gated protocols have been reported to be less than 1 mSv in studies using low peak kilovoltage and low milliamperes per kilogram. On the contrary, retrospective ECG-gated scanning yields higher radiation doses, estimated to be around 3–10 mSv, even with the low-dose technique [5–10]. Another technique that may be used to lower the radiation dose for the patient is adaptive statistical iterative reconstruction, a unique CT reconstruction algorithm with matrix algebra used to selectively identify and subtract noise from the image. The result is less noise or the same amount of noise with less radiation [8–11].

CT Data Postprocessing and Analysis

At our institution, all images have a reconstruction section thickness of 0.625 mm and a section interval of 0.625 mm with use of a small cardiac field of view. The lung window is reconstructed at a 2.5-mm section. All images obtained are transferred to an external workstation, where they are reconstructed with multiplanar reformation, volume rendering, and maximum intensity projections. The protocol parameters used at our institution are described in detail in Table 2.2.

Table 2.2 MDCT cardiac CTA prottvocols in infants for a 64-slice GE scanner

	ECG-gated scanning technique	
Parameter	Retrospective	Prospective
Contrast	Iodinated contrast medium (iopamidol, 300 mg/ml) is used at 1 ml/lb of body weight with injection speed of 0.7 ml/s	Iodinated contrast medium (iopamidol, 300 mg/ml) is used at 1 ml/lb of body weight with injection speed of 0.7 ml/s
Peak kilovoltage	80	80
Milliamperes	weight based protocol	weight based protocol
R-R interval	Entire interval	50–75 %
Pitch	0.2–0.24	No pitch
Padding	None	175 ms
Rotation, *sec*	0.35	0.35
Collimation, *mm*	0.6	0.6
Slice thickness, *mm*	0.625	0.625
Field of view	Small cardiac	Small cardiac

References

1. Jin KN, Park EA, Shin CI, Lee W, Chung JW, Park JH. Retrospective versus prospective ECG-gated dual-source CT in pediatric patients with congenital heart diseases: comparison of image quality and radiation dose. Int J Cardiovasc Imaging. 2010;26 Suppl 1:63–73.
2. Hollingsworth CL, Yoshizumi TT, Frush DP, Chan FP, Toncheva G, Nguyen G, et al. Pediatric cardiac-gated CT angiography: assessment of radiation dose. AJR Am J Roentgenol. 2007;189(1):12–8.
3. Paul JF, Rohnean A, Elfassy E, Sigal-Cinqualbre A. Radiation dose for thoracic and coronary step-and-shoot CT using a 128-slice dual-source machine in infants and small children with congenital heart disease. Pediatr Radiol. 2011;41(2):244–9.
4. Paul JF, Rohnean A, Sigal-Cinqualbre A. Multidetector CT for congenital heart patients: what a paediatric radiologist should know. Pediatr Radiol. 2010;40(6): 869–75.
5. Hirai N, Horiguchi J, Fujioka C, Kiguchi M, Yamamoto H, Matsuura N, et al. Prospective versus retrospective ECG-gated 64 detector coronary CT angiography: assessment of image quality, stenosis, and radiation dose. Radiology. 2008;248(2):424–30.
6. Kuettner A, Gehann B, Spolnik J, Koch A, Achenbach S, Weyand M, et al. Strategies for dose-optimized imaging in pediatric cardiac dual source CT. Rofo. 2009;181(4):339–48.
7. Huang B, Law MW, Mak HK, Kwok SP, Khong PL. Pediatric 64-MDCT coronary angiography with ECG-modulated tube current: radiation dose and cancer risk. AJR Am J Roentgenol. 2009;193(2):539–44.
8. Al-Mousily F, Shifrin RY, Fricker FJ, Feranec N, Quinn NS, Chandran A. Use of 320-detector computed tomographic angiography for infants and young children with congenital heart disease. Pediatr Cardiol. 2011;32(4):426–32.
9. Pages J, Buls N, Osteaux M. CT doses in children: a multicentre study. Br J Radiol. 2003;76(911):803–11.
10. Deak PD, Smal Y, Kalender WA. Multisection CT protocols: sex- and age-specific conversion factors used to determine effective dose from dose-length product. Radiology. 2010;257(1):158–66.
11. Li X, Samei E, Segars WP, Sturgeon GM, Colsher JG, Frush DP. Patient-specific radiation dose and cancer risk for pediatric chest CT. Radiology. 2011;259(3):862–74.

Advanced Postprocessing of Cardiac CTA

3

Randy Ray Richardson

Functional Evaluation of Cardiac CTA

Commercially available workstations have software packages to provide volumetric analysis for cardiac CTA. In children, it is best to obtain the data prospectively to reduce radiation exposure. The rapid heart rate of infants results in data and phases of a larger portion of the cardiac cycle than in adults with the same amount of padding. End-systolic and end-diastolic volumes are obtained easily for both right and left ventricles. The typical part of the phase to obtain the end-diastolic data is at 85–90 % of the cardiac cycle. The typical part of the phase to obtain the end-systolic data is at 45–55 % of the cardiac cycle. Once volumes have been determined for end systole and end diastole, the ejection fraction and stroke volume can be calculated and provided as part of the report. It is helpful to divide the end-diastolic and end-systolic volumes by body surface area to provide indexed volumes. Indexed volumes are obtained by dividing the gross end-diastolic and end-systolic volume of the right and left ventricles by the body surface area (Figs. 3.1, 3.2 and Table 3.1).

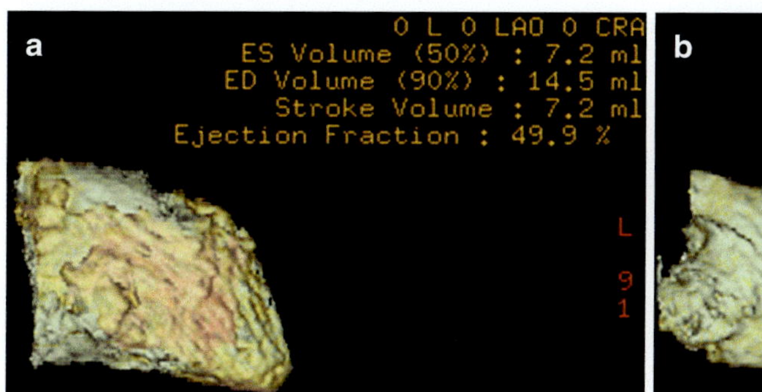

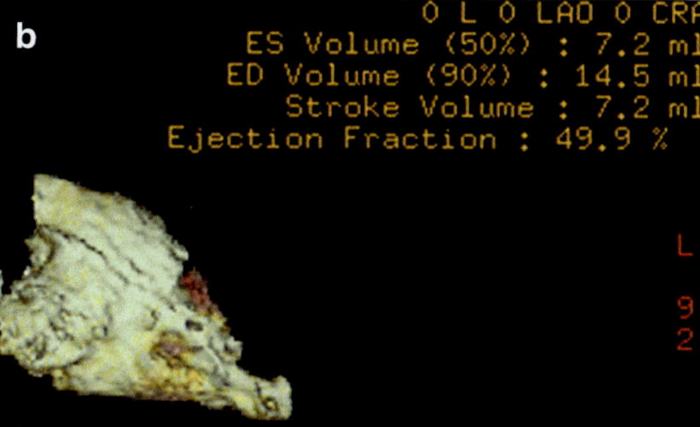

Fig. 3.1 End-systolic (**a**) and end-diastolic (**b**) volume of the right ventricle. Evaluation of the data is provided in Table 3.1

R.R. Richardson, MD
Department of Radiology,
St. Joseph's Hospital and Medical Center,
Creighton University School of Medicine,
West Thomas Rd 350, 85013 Phoenix, AZ, USA
e-mail: randy.richardson2@chw.edu,
randy.richardson2@dignityhealth.org

R.R. Richardson, *Atlas of Pediatric Cardiac CTA*,
DOI 10.1007/978-1-4614-0088-2_3, © Springer Science+Business Media New York 2013

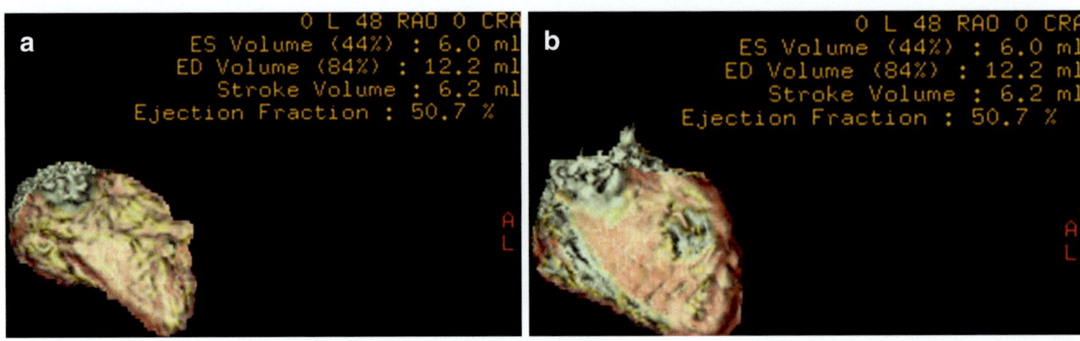

Fig. 3.2 End-systolic (**a**) and end-diastolic (**b**) volume of the left ventricle. Evaluation of the data is provided in Table 3.1

Table 3.1 Functional cardiac CTA calculations

RV and LV parameters	Gross volume, *mL*	BSA, m^2	Gross volume ÷ BSA = volume index, mL/m^2	Normal volume index range, mL/m^2 [a]	Ejection fraction, % (*range*, %)
RV end-systolic	7.2	0.2	36	19–30	–
RV end-diastolic	14.5	0.2	72.5	62–88	–
RV stroke volume	7.2	–	–	No normal indexed values	–
RV	–	–	–	–	49.9 (40–60)
LV end-systolic	6.0	0.2	30	17–37	–
LV end-diastolic	12.2	0.2	61	50–84	–
LV stroke volume	6.2	0.2	31	30–65	–
LV	–	–	–	–	50.7 (50–70)

BSA body surface area, *LV* left ventricular, *RV* right ventricular
[a]Normal values are taken from GE report card postprocessing software

Volumetric Analysis of Blood Flow

CT postprocessing of pulmonary vasculature may be performed using a commercially available three-dimensional (3D) workstation. The pulmonary vasculature (pulmonary arteries and veins) is grown out with the aid of an automated vessel selection tool. The arterial pulmonary circulation is grown out proximally from the pulmonary valve and distally as far as the smallest opacified vessel. The venous pulmonary circulation is grown out similarly from the left atrial ostia to the smallest opacified vessel. The automated selection is then reviewed for any nonvascular components, which are cut out from the selection manually. Once the pulmonary vasculature has been grown out fully, the left and right pulmonary circulations are divided by hand. The division point for each side occurs at the origin of the right main and left main pulmonary artery. The main pulmonary artery is then excluded. Once the selections are complete, the pulmonary vascular volume is calculated using the workstation volume quantification software. This process may be better appreciated in Fig. 3.3.

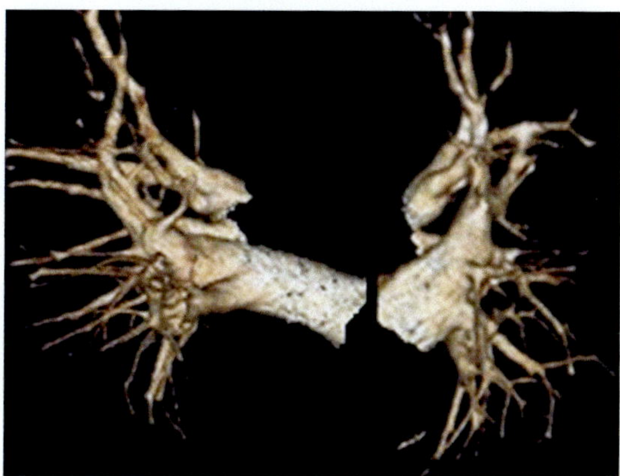

Fig. 3.3 Right and left pulmonary arteries and veins grown out for volumetric analysis of blood flow. The percent flow to the right is 81.006 (total right volume) divided by 135.992 (total combined volume), which equals 60 % volumetric flow to the right lung. Using the same calculation for the left (54.986/135.992), there is 40 % volumetric flow to the left lung

Statistical Analysis

The right pulmonary blood volume percentage is obtained by dividing the pulmonary blood volume from the right side by the total pulmonary blood volume from both the right and left sides. Thc same calculation is performed to determine the percentage of pulmonary blood volume on the left.

Standardized Color Coding

Most of the 3D images in this book are color coded. A standardized 3D color-coding scheme is used to help communicate findings. This technique has been used to improve the understanding of complex anatomy. Using the images in conferences and consultations allows viewers to quickly and efficiently understand the anatomy. This has been particularly useful for surgeons, cardiologists, residents, nurses, students, and other health care providers. Three-dimensional images are particularly useful when demonstrating the anatomy in patients with complex congenital heart disease. This color scheme is derived from a palette of commonly used colors currently associated with the arterial and venous structures, such as red for the aorta, blue for the pulmonary veins, and so forth.

Currently, we use a commercially available workstation to segment the anatomic components. This process typically takes 20 min to perform. Once the anatomic structures are segmented, colors are assigned to the segmented anatomy using the color coding scheme shown in Figs. 3.4, 3.5, 3.6, 3.7, and 3.8.

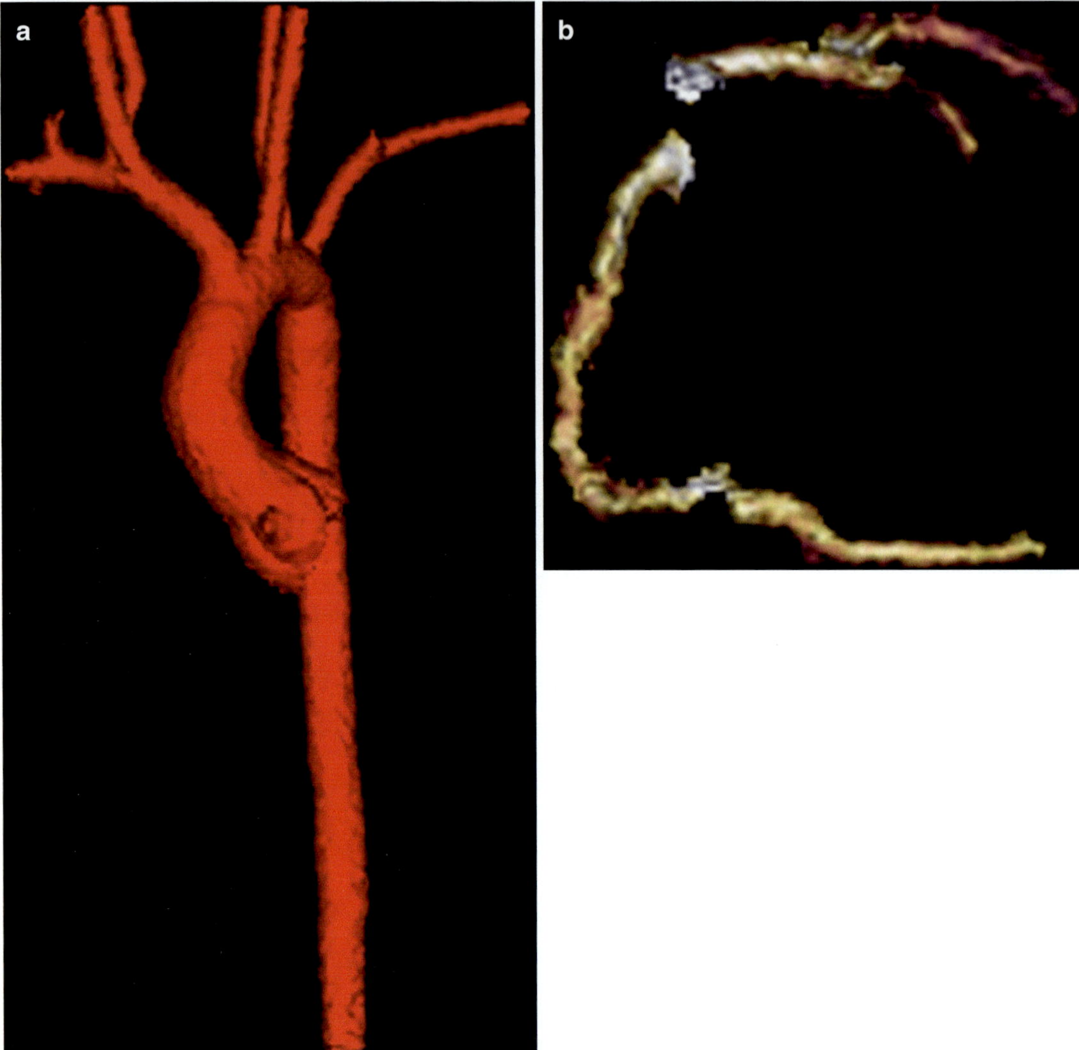

Fig. 3.4 (**a**) *Red* is used for the aorta. (**b**) The coronary arteries are a neutral color

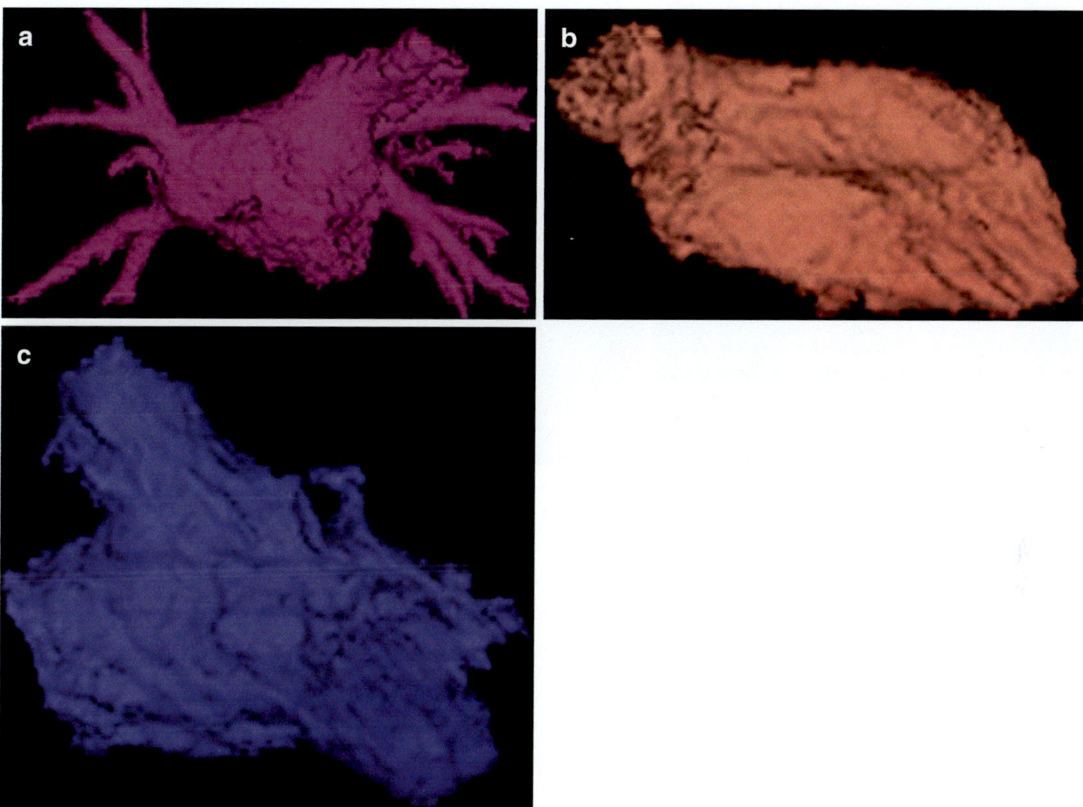

Fig. 3.5 *Pink* is used for the pulmonary veins (**a**), *salmon* for the left ventricle (**b**), and *violet* for the right ventricle (**c**)

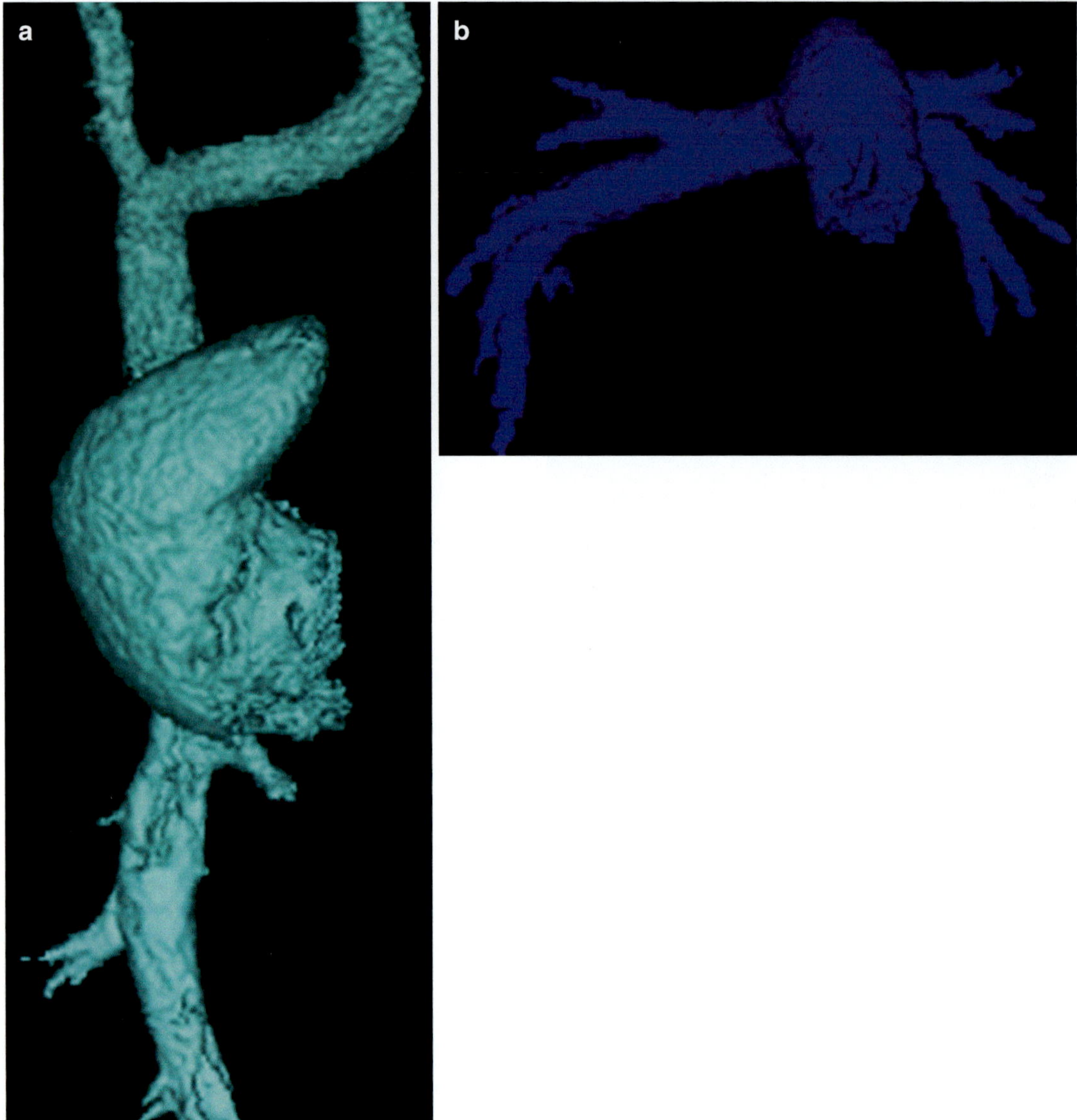

Fig. 3.6 (**a**) The right atrium and systemic veins are colored *light blue*. (**b**) The pulmonary artery appears *dark blue*

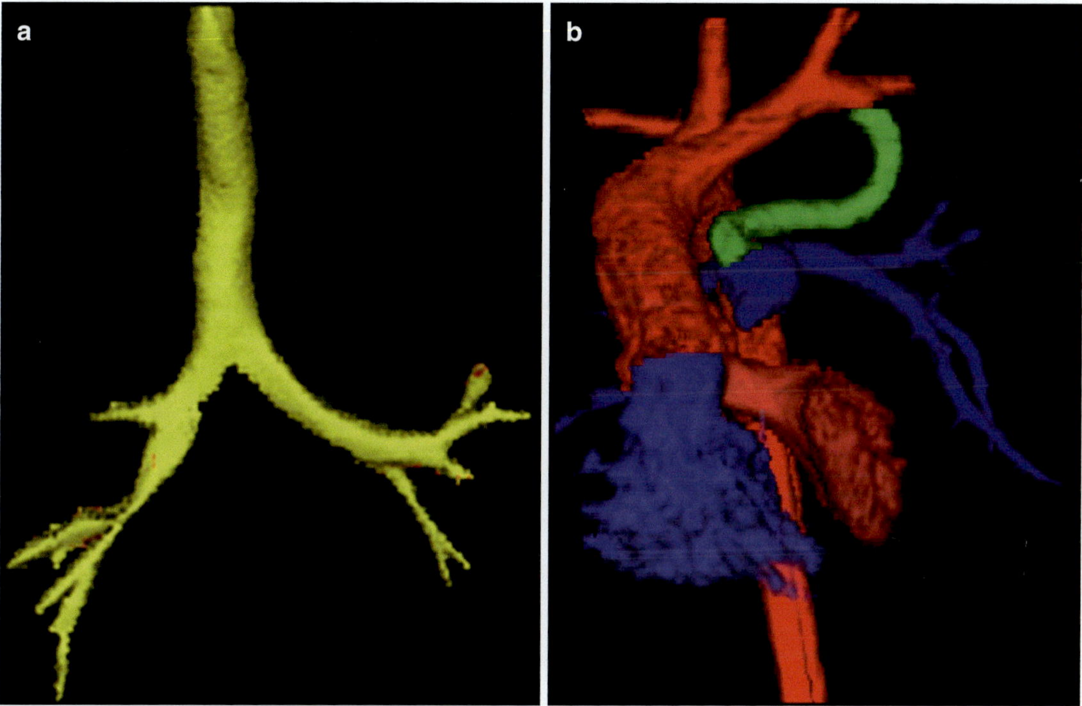

Fig. 3.7 (**a**) The trachea is colored *yellow*. (**b**) Surgically created shunts and patent ductus arteriosus are *green*

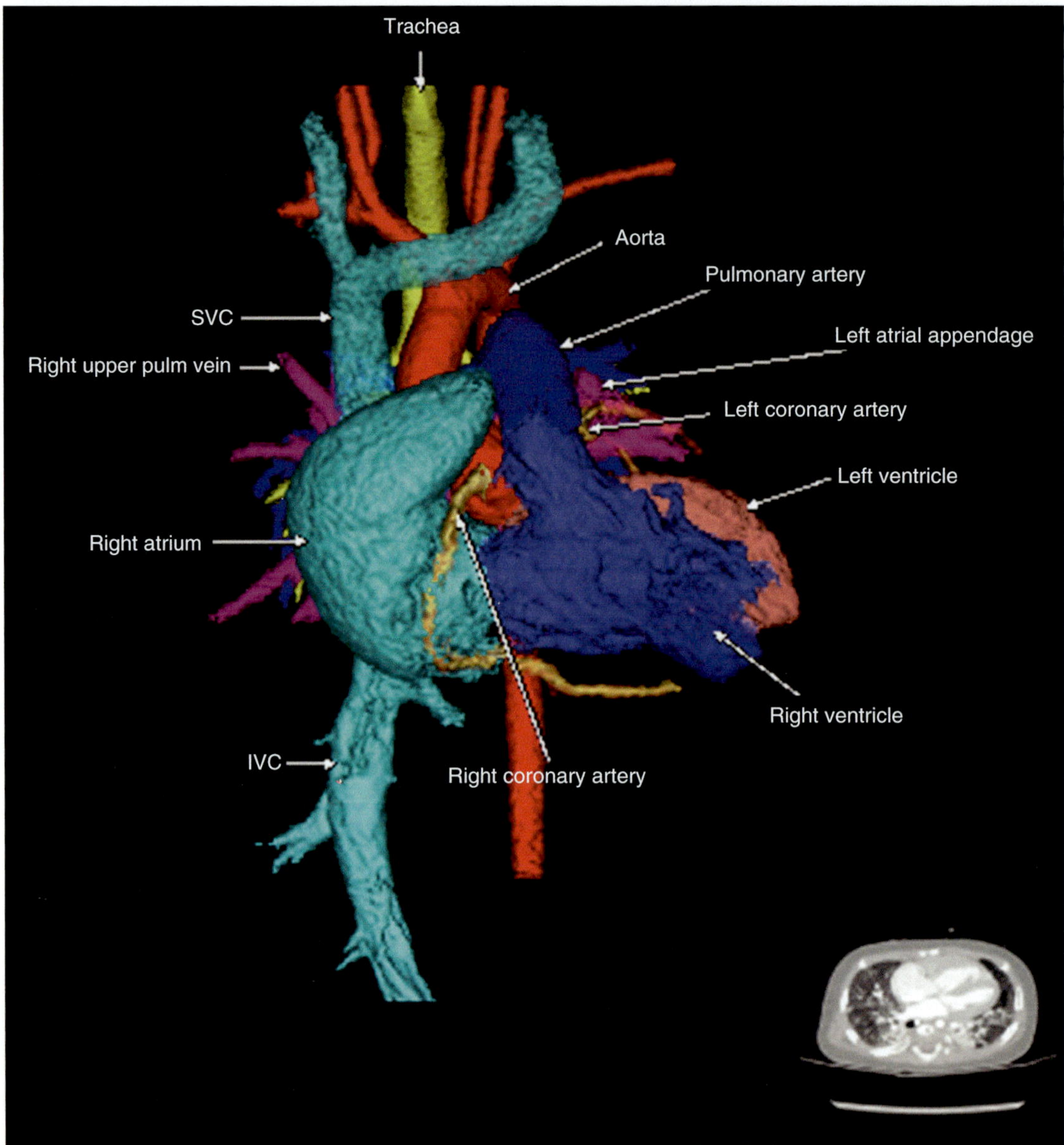

Fig. 3.8 The individual structures are then pieced together to create the full color-coded 3D model, which can be sent to the picture archiving and communication system so health care providers can understand the patient's anatomy. *IVC* inferior vena cava, *SVC* superior vena cava

Color-Coded Resin Models

Once the segmentation and coloring of the models are complete, the data exist to create an actual 3D resin model of the anatomy. A 3D rapid prototyping machine may be used to create models of the heart. These models are to scale and may be sterilized and used in the operating room (Fig. 3.9).

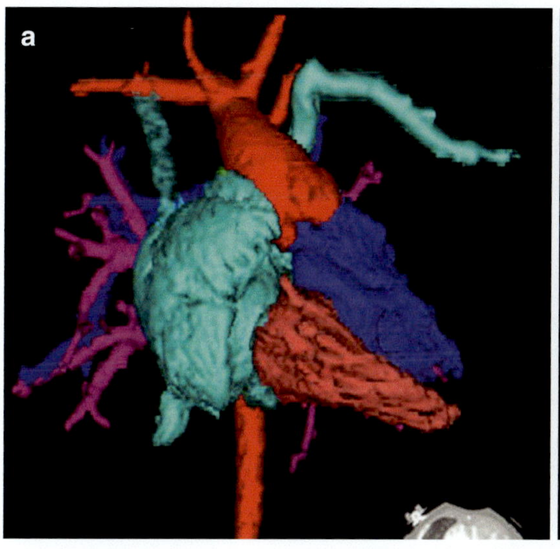

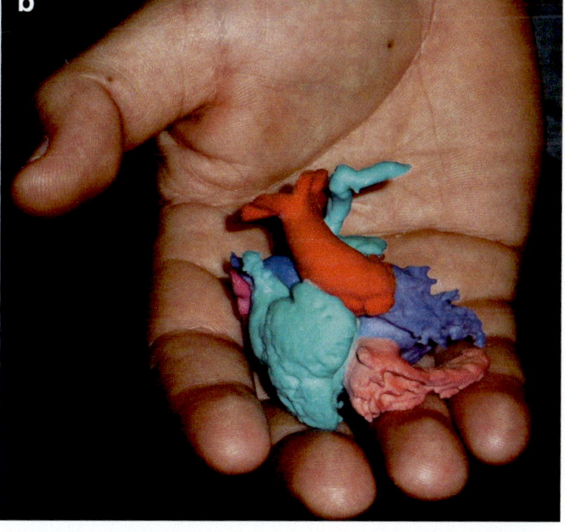

Fig. 3.9 A frontal projection color-coded 3D model (**a**) and a 3D resin model (**b**) of the same anatomy. In the future, these color-coded models may be created using synthetic materials to provide a realistic texture of the patient's anatomic defects. This might allow for improved training and the sharing of complex surgical and angiographic techniques for patients with complex congenital heart disease

Systematic Evaluation of Cardiac CTA

4

Randy Ray Richardson and Ernerio T. Alboliras

Cardiac CT evaluation requires a systematic approach to evaluate the complex anatomy in congenital heart patients. We suggest the following outline to assess these patients:

1. Systemic and pulmonary veins, atria, and atrioventricular (AV) valves. Start by evaluating the atria and AV valves of the heart and the veins returning blood to the heart. Look for the following:
   (a) A right superior vena cava (SVC) and inferior vena cava (IVC)
   (b) A left SVC. Check to determine whether this is solitary or if there is a bilateral SVC with or without a crossing brachiocephalic vein. Also, determine the atrial connection of the SVC; check whether it connects directly to the atrium, or if there is a connection into a coronary sinus.
   (c) Atrial connection of the IVC. Rarely, it may be bilateral or cross the spine to connect with the contralateral atrium.
   (d) Pulmonary venous return. Pulmonary veins may return blood anomalously to the systemic circulation, such as the IVC, SVC, or brachiocephalic vein. Anomalous pulmonary venous return may be partial or total depending on whether all or part of the blood goes to the systemic circulation. It also may be mixed anomalous drainage. Check for a detailed connection of each pulmonary vein.
   (e) Defects in the atrial septum. Types of defects include secundum, primum, patent foramen ovale, and sinus venosus defect. These may be difficult to see and may require viewing different phases of the scan to optimize visualization. It is helpful to correlate these images with echocardiographic examinations.
   (f) Relative size and appearance of the atria and atrial appendages.
   (g) AV valve anomalies, including atresia, stenosis, dysplasia (a dysplastic septal leaflet of the tricuspid valve is seen with Ebstein's anomaly), a common AV valve, and thickening of the valves. Valve sizes should be provided. Subtle vegetations may be seen. Correlation with echocardiography may be helpful when subtle findings are suspected.
2. Ventricles
   (a) Distinguish the morphologic right ventricle (RV) from the left ventricle (LV). The RV typically has a more trabeculated septal surface than the LV; it also has a more pyramidal shape, with a moderator band at its apex. The LV has an ellipsoid shape and a smoother septal surface. The RV outflow tract or infundibulum is muscle bound and typically not in fibrous continuity with the tricuspid valve.

R.R. Richardson, MD (✉)
Department of Radiology,
St. Joseph's Hospital and Medical Center,
Creighton University School of Medicine,
West Thomas Rd 350, 85013 Phoenix, AZ, USA
e-mail: randy.richardson2@chw.edu,
randy.richardson2@dignityhealth.org

E.T. Alboliras, MD
Children's Heart Center,
Phoenix Children's Hospital,
Phoenix, AZ, USA

R.R. Richardson, *Atlas of Pediatric Cardiac CTA*,
DOI 10.1007/978-1-4614-0088-2_4, © Springer Science+Business Media New York 2013

(b) Look for ventricular septal defects. These are seen most commonly in the perimembranous region of the ventricular septum but also may be observed in the muscular portion of the septum, subvalvular region, or posteriorly along the septum in patients with AV septal defects.
(c) Evaluate ventricular size, motion, and function if sufficient data are available.
(d) Look for an abnormally thickened myocardium, which may be a primary or secondary abnormality and may lead to outflow tract obstruction.

3. Great vessels. Assess the following:
   (a) Outflow tracts. They may be switched, narrowed, absent, or aneurysmal.
   (b) Aorta
      (i) It may be discontinuous (interruption of the aortic arch), stenotic in patients with coarctation of the aorta or supravalvular aortic stenosis, or hypoplastic.
      (ii) Identify whether the arch is on the left or right, and determine the number and location of vessels arising from the arch. Vascular rings, such as a double arch or right arch with an aberrant left subclavian artery, may cause airway obstruction.
      (iii) Look for aortopulmonary collaterals. These typically are seen along the descending aorta but may arise from the arch or great vessels.
      (iv) Measure the size and caliber of the aorta at the aortic annulus, sinus of Valsalva, sinotubular junction, transverse arch, and descending aorta. Comparison with normative data (z-score) may be helpful.
   (c) Pulmonary arteries
      (i) They may be atretic, hypoplastic, or anomalous. Determine the origin and course of the pulmonary arteries. Some pulmonary arteries may arise from the aorta, patent ductus arteriosus (PDA) or the other pulmonary artery (in pulmonary sling, the left pulmonary artery arises from the right and courses around the trachea, often causing tracheal or bronchial stenosis).
      (ii) Evaluate the size of the main pulmonary artery and the right and left proximal and distal pulmonary arteries.
      (iii) Look for other vessels connected to the pulmonary arteries, such as a PDA. Aortopulmonary collaterals may be connected to the pulmonary artries or may supply the lung directly.
   (d) PDA (patent ductus arteriosus)
      (i) PDA typically originates from the undersurface of the descending aorta or left brachiocephalic/subclavian artery but rarely may have other anomalous origins and may be bilateral, with one part arising from the aorta and the other from the brachiocephalic artery.
      (ii) It may be large and tortuous, especially in patients with complex congenital heart disease. A diverticulum may be seen at the origin of the ductus (Kommerell's diverticulum). Look for mass effect from the enlarged PDA on other adjacent structures (especially the trachea and bronchi).
      (iii) Later in life, a calcification often is seen in the region of the ligamentum arteriosum that forms when the ductus closes.
4. Coronary arteries
   (a) Evaluate the origin, number, course, and termination of the coronary arteries. Notify the surgeon of an anomalous course, especially if it crosses an outflow tract.
   (b) Rarely, a coronary artery may arise from the pulmonary artery, such as in anomalous left coronary artery from the pulmonary artery (ALCAPA).
   (c) An increased caliber of the coronary arteries in a newborn may suggest a fistulous communication with a low-pressure system, such as the RV or pulmonary artery.
5. Lungs and airways
   (a) Congenital airway anomalies are more common in patients with congenital heart

disease. Congenital stenosis and bilateral left- or right-sidedness is common in patients with asplenia- or polysplenia-type heterotaxies.
   (b) Look specifically for a right upper lobe (pig) bronchus, especially in patients with chronic right upper lobe collapse.
   (c) Tracheobronchomalacia is common in congenital heart patients. A narrowed horseshoe-like appearance of the airway may be seen on CT.
   (d) Extrinsic airway compression is very common in patients with complex congenital heart disease. Look for vascular rings, pulmonary sling, and dilated structures compressing the airway.
6. Situs and cardiac position
   (a) Designate each patient as situs solitus (normal), situs inversus (reversed), or situs ambiguous (indeterminate).
   (b) Situs usually is determined by the sidedness of the liver, stomach, spleen, right atrial appendages, IVC, and cardiac position. In addition, the anatomy of the tracheobronchial tree and the relationship of the right and left mainstem bronchi with respect to the right and left pulmonary artery are important hallmarks.
   (c) Thc normal heart is in levocardia (at the left chest), with the apex pointed to the left. Dextrocardia occurs when the heart is in the right side of the chest. In this case, the apex may point to the right or to the left. In mesocardia, the heart is in the midline, with the apex pointed inferiorly, or is difficult to ascertain.
   (d) If the aforementioned structures are positioned normally, they are in *situs solitus*. If the structures are reversed, they are in *situs inversus*. If there is a combination of both positions, the structures are in *situs ambiguous*.
   (e) The presence of situs ambiguous may be a hallmark of asplenia and polysplenia heterotaxy syndrome
7. Common surgical procedures in patients with congenital heart disease. When dealing with congenital heart disease, it is vital to understand the basic terminology regarding postoperative shunts, procedures, and surgeries.

5 Evaluation of the Atria, Atrioventricular Valves, and Veins

Randy Ray Richardson and Andrew Duarte

One should begin cardiac CT evaluation by assessing the atria, the systemic and pulmonary veins draining to them, and the atrioventricular (AV) valves. Examine the following:

(a) Anatomy of the right atrium, left atrium, or a common atrium. Assess whether there is atrial inversion, and determine the size of each atrium (hypoplasia or dilatation).
(b) Atrial appendages. The right atrial appendage is triangular and directed anteriorly and superiorly, whereas the left atrial appendage is tongue shaped and directed laterally (leftward). In some complex heart defects, the atrial appendages may be difficult to identify. Look for an abnormal right-sided or a left-sided juxtaposition of the atrial appendages.
(c) Superior vena cava (SVC) and inferior vena cava (IVC). The normal SVC inserts into the right-sided morphologic right atrium, whereas the IVC inserts into the medial, posterior, and inferior aspect of the right atrium. The hepatic veins communicate with the IVC. A left SVC may be present with or without a crossing brachiocephalic vein that connects to a right SVC. It is important to determine whether the left SVC empties into a coronary sinus that then drains to the right atrium, or whether it empties directly into the left atrium.
(d) Pulmonary veins. Typically, there are four pulmonary veins connecting to the morphologic left atrium. However, sometimes two veins may fuse into one before joining the left atrium, or multiple pulmonary veins may drain to one side before they reach the left atrium. Pulmonary veins that drain anomalously should be identified—one, some, or all of the pulmonary veins may drain to the IVC, hepatic vein, SVC, or brachiocephalic vein. Total anomalous pulmonary venous connection occurs if all pulmonary veins drain anomalously either together through a common pulmonary venous chamber or through mixed or different locations. A common association of a right upper or lower partial anomalous pulmonary vein on the right vein is the presence of a sinus venosus type of atrial septal defect (ASD). A partial anomalous pulmonary venous connection of all or most of the right-sided pulmonary veins is seen in scimitar syndrome, in which the anomalous connection is into the IVC. This is associated with a hypoplastic right lung and right pulmonary artery as well as systemic arterial supply to the right lower lobe.
(e) Atrial septum. Defects in the atrial septum may be difficult to see and may require assessment of different phases of the scan to

R.R. Richardson, MD (✉)
Department of Radiology,
St. Joseph's Hospital and Medical Center,
Creighton University School of Medicine,
West Thomas Rd 350, 85013 Phoenix, AZ, USA
e-mail: randy.richardson2@chw.edu,
randy.richardson2@dignityhealth.org

A. Duarte, MD
Radiology Residency Program,
St. Joseph's Hospital and Medical Center,
Phoenix, AZ, USA

R.R. Richardson, *Atlas of Pediatric Cardiac CTA*,
DOI 10.1007/978-1-4614-0088-2_5, © Springer Science+Business Media New York 2013

optimize visualization. Echocardiography provides optimal visualization of the type, size, extent, and number of ASDs.

(f) AV valves. There are two AV valves: the tricuspid valve, which drains into the right ventricle, and the mitral valve, which drains into the left ventricle. Anomalies include dilatation, hypoplasia, dysplasia, atresia, overriding annulus, straddling chordae, common AV valve, and the presence of Ebstein's malformation. Ebstein's anomaly, a spectrum of tricuspid anomaly that occurs when there is apical displacement of the septal leaflet and dysplasia of the posterior leaflet, and when the anterior leaflet becomes sail-like, with some degree of tethering to the right ventricular (RV) wall. This results in atrialization of a portion of the right ventricle and, rarely, obstruction of the RV outflow tract.

Normal Anatomy of the Atria and Veins

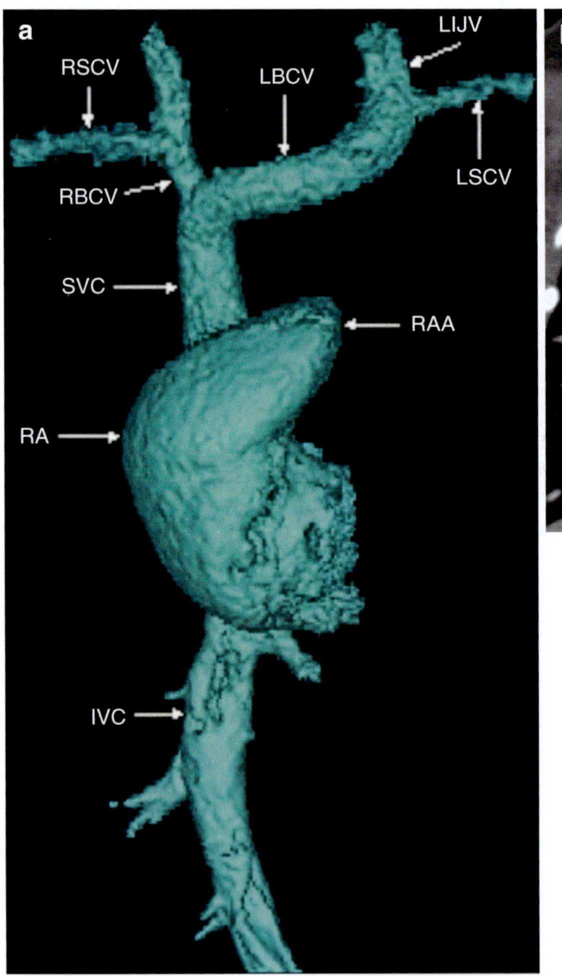

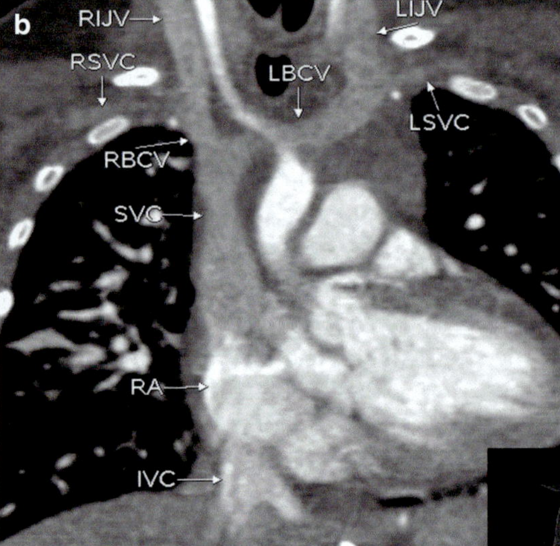

Fig. 5.1 Frontal projection three-dimensional (3D) model (**a**) and coronal maximum-intensity projection (MIP) image (**b**) from a cardiac CTA shows normal anatomy of the normal right-sided SVC (*RSVC*) draining the left brachiocephalic vein (*LBCV*) and right brachiocephalic vein (*RBCV*) into the right atrium (*RA*). Note the typical triangular shape of the right atrial appendage (*RAA*). *LIJV* left internal jugular vein, *LSCV* left subclavian vein, *LSVC* left SVC, *RIJV* right internal jugular vein, *RSCV* right subclavian vein, *IVC* inferior vena cava, *SVC* superior vena cava

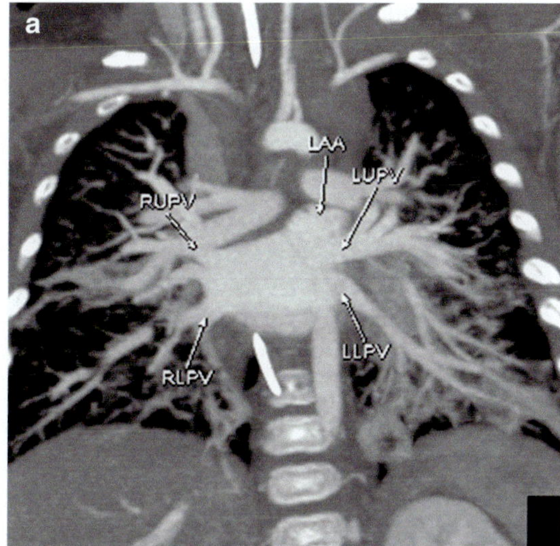

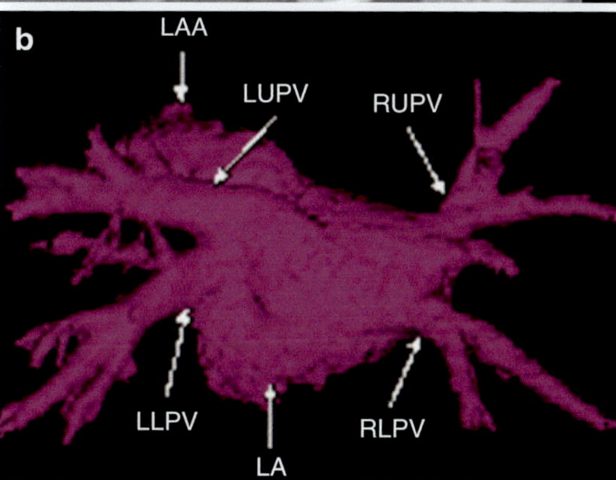

Fig. 5.2 Coronal MIP (**a**) and posterior projection 3D color-coded (**b**) images from a cardiac CTA scan demonstrating normal anatomy, with right and left upper and lower pulmonary veins (*RUPV* right upper pulmonary vein, *LUPV* left upper pulmonary vein, *RLPV* right lower pulmonary vein, *LLPV* left lower pulmonary vein, respectively) draining to the left atrium (*LA*) and a normal-appearing left atrial appendage (*LAA*). Note the elongated, tongue-like appearance of the left atrial appendage

Left Superior Vena Cava

Left SVC is a common variant, especially in patients with congenital heart disease. It is important to make this finding for presurgical planning in patients undergoing SVC shunts so that there is no collateral flow around the shunt. In most instances, there is duplicated SVC physiology, with the left SVC draining blood from the left

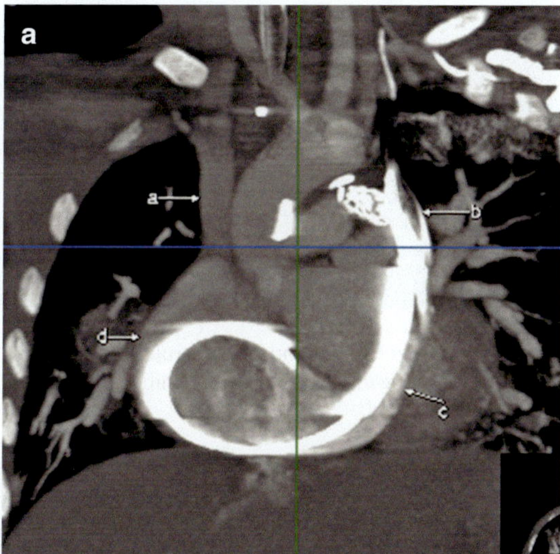

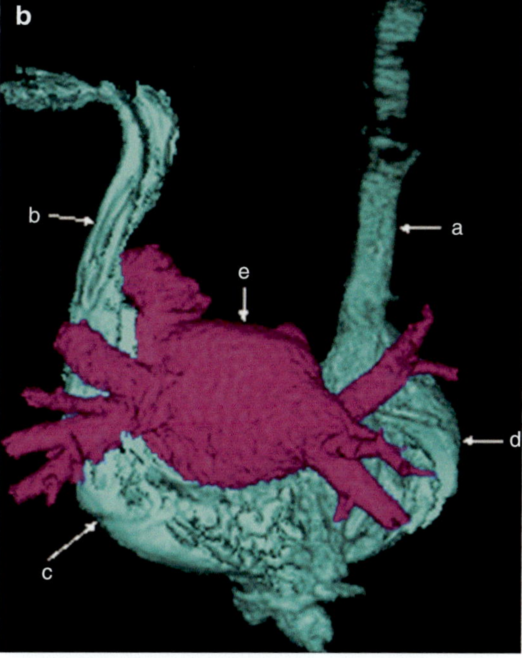

Fig. 5.3 Coronal MIP (**a**) and posterior projection color-coded 3D (**b**) images from a cardiac CT scan showing a left SVC (*b*) draining to the right atrium (*d*) via a large coronary sinus (*c*). Notice the distal right SVC (*a*) draining normally into the right atrium (*d*). Notice the elongated left atrial appendage adjacent to the left SVC (*b*)

internal jugular and left subclavian veins and the right-sided systemic veins draining to a right SVC. In patients with atrial inversion that may be associated with heterotaxy syndrome, the left SVC may be the morphologic right SVC.

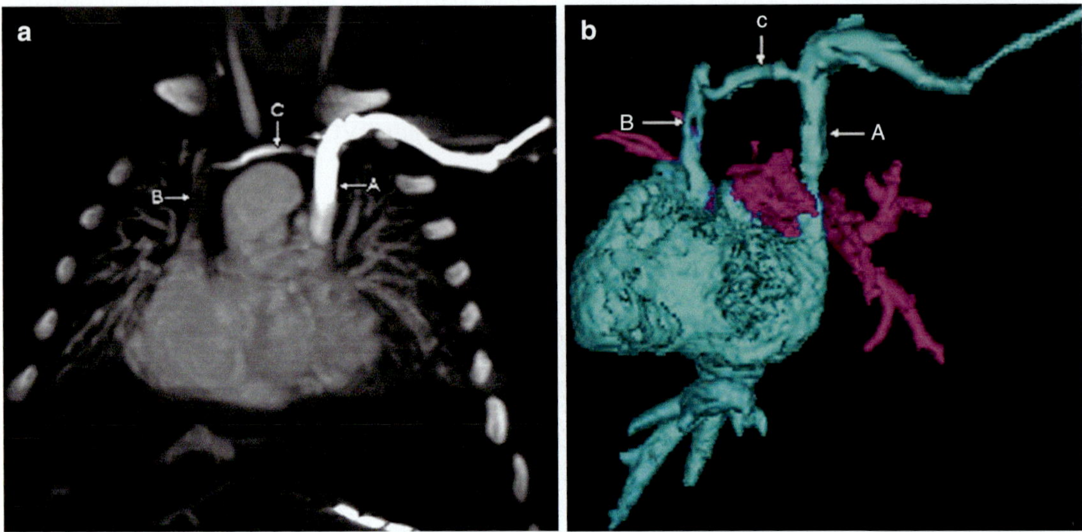

Fig. 5.4 Coronal MIP (**a**) and frontal projection color-coded 3D (**b**) images from a cardiac CT scan showing a right (*B*) and left (*A*) SVC with a connecting brachiocephalic vein (*C*).

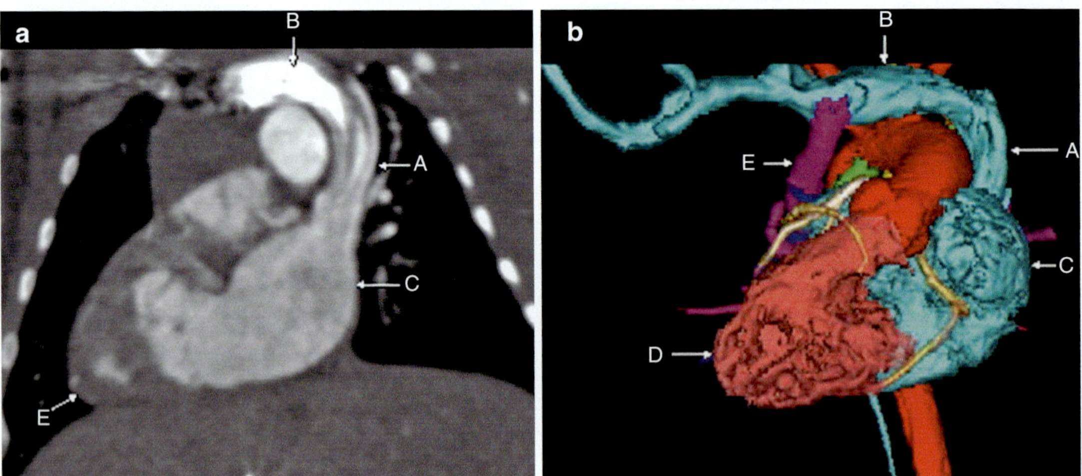

Fig. 5.5 Coronal MIP (**a**) and frontal projection color-coded 3D (**b**) images from a cardiac CT scan showing a right brachiocephalic vein (*B*) emptying into a left SVC (*A*) draining to the left atrium (*C*) in a patient with situs inversus. This may be associated with other congenital anomalies, such as total anomalous pulmonary venous return (TAPVR). In this case, a right-sided vertical vein (*E* in **b**) drains blood from the pulmonary veins (*pink*) to the brachiocephalic vein (*B*). Also notice that the apex of the heart is on the right, consistent with dextrocardia and known situs ambiguous in a patient with heterotaxy syndrome

Partial Anomalous Pulmonary Venous Return

Partial anomalous pulmonary venous return (PAPVR) has the following characteristics:

1. One or more, but not all, pulmonary veins flow to a systemic vein
2. One pulmonary lobe typically is involved, although the whole lung may be involved
3. It typically is asymptomatic
4. If symptoms occur, they usually are the result of right heart overload from increased volume
5. It is associated with sinus venosus ASD and scimitar syndrome.

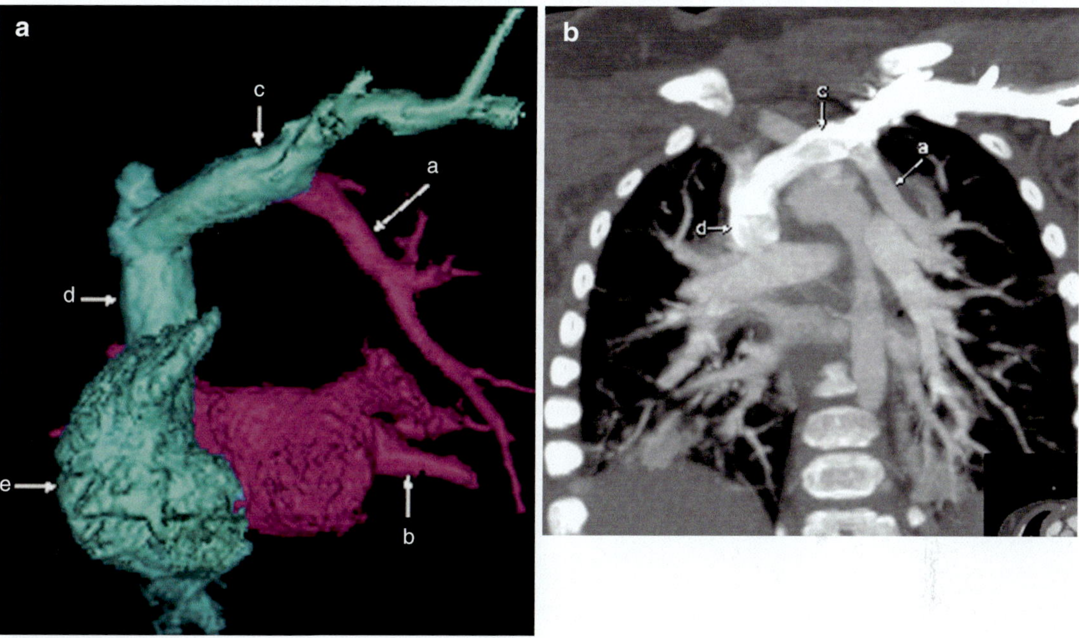

Fig. 5.6 Frontal projection 3D color-coded (**a**) and coronal MIP (**b**) images demonstrating a left upper lobe pulmonary vein (*a*) anomalously draining to the left brachiocephalic vein (*c*). The SVC (*d*) and right atrium (*e*) are mildly prominent. Notice that there is normal drainage of the left lower lobe pulmonary vein (*b*) to the left atrium

Supracardiac TAPVR Type 1

In the most common type of supracardiac TAPVR, the pulmonary veins form a common chamber connected to a vertical vein that in turn drains to the left brachiocephalic vein, which connects to the SVC. Occasionally, supracardiac TAPVR may connect to the right-sided SVC through a vessel that crosses the midline. Obstruction to the pulmonary venous blood flow may occur as the vertical vein crosses the bronchi or at its entry to the systemic vein. All types of TAPVR are left-to-right shunts that form obligatory right-to-left shunts through an ASD or patent ductus arteriosus after mixing with systemic venous blood. Thus, patients are cyanotic. This lesion may be isolated or associated with complex congenital heart disease and heterotaxy syndromes. All total anomalous pulmonary venous connections (TAPVCs) result in increased pulmonary blood flow.

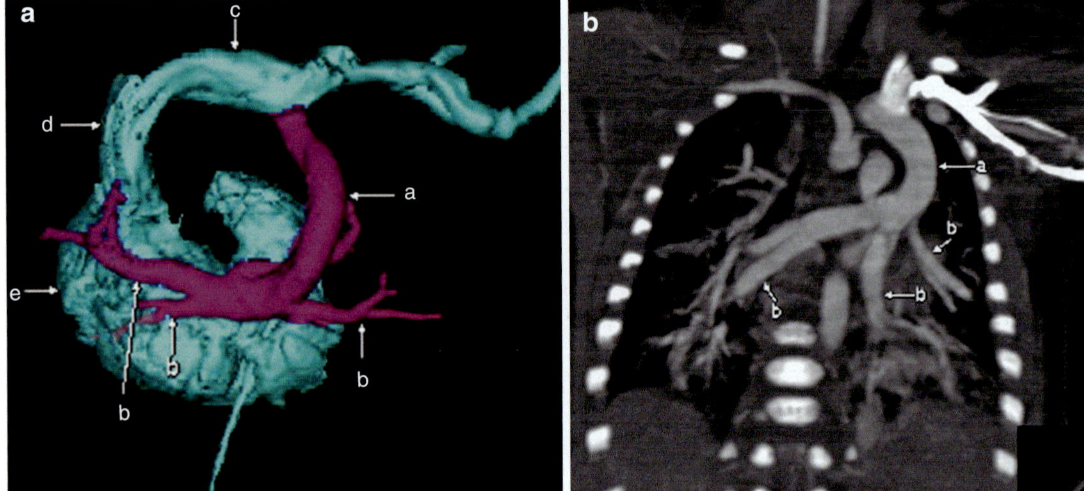

Fig. 5.7 Posterior projection 3D color model from CTA (**a**) and coronal MIP (**b**) images demonstrating multiple pulmonary veins (*b*) draining to a vertical vein (*a*), which connects to the brachiocephalic vein (*c*) and to the SVC (*d*) back to the systemic atrium (*e*)

Intracardiac TAPVR

Intracardiac TAPVR is also a left-to-right shunt that requires an obligatory right-to-left shunt through an ASD for adequate systemic cardiac output. Thus, patients may appear cyanotic. TAPVC draining into the coronary sinus is the second most common type of TAPVC; direct right atrial drainage is less common. Pulmonary venous obstruction is unusual.

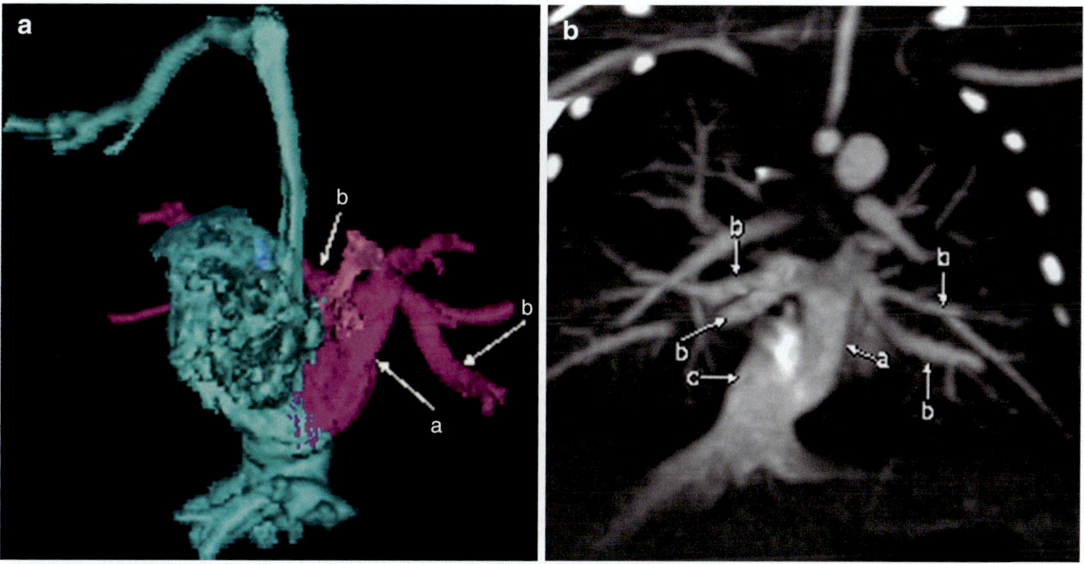

Fig. 5.8 Anterior projection 3D color model (**a**) and coronal MIP image (**b**) showing multiple pulmonary veins (*b*) draining directly to the coronary sinus (*a*) back to the right atrium (*c*)

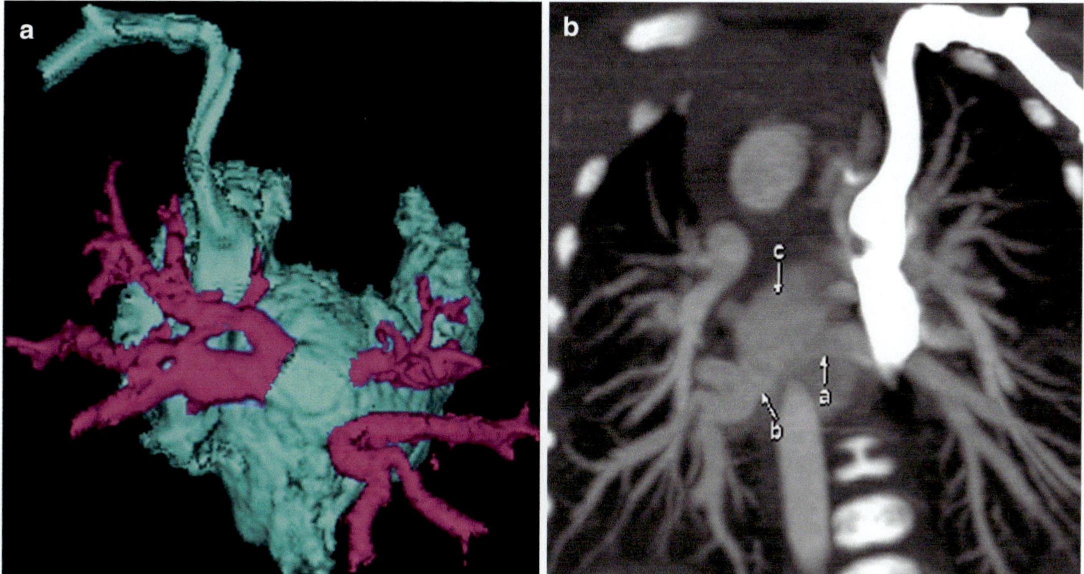

Fig. 5.9 Posterior projection 3D color model (**a**) and coronal MIP image (**b**) demonstrating multiple pulmonary veins (*pink*, *a* and *b*) draining directly to the right atrium (*light blue*, *c*) in a patient with TAPVR

Infracardiac TAPVR

In infracardiac TAPVR, the pulmonary veins drain to a vertical vein that empties into the IVC, portal vein, or hepatic veins. This type of TAPVR is associated with congestive heart failure due to obstruction of the pulmonary venous drainage. Pulmonary venous obstruction also may result from narrowing of the vertical vein as it passes through the diaphragm, narrowing at the insertion into the intrahepatic vessel, with blood having to pass through the hepatic capillary bed (if the insertion is to a portal vein) or a hypoplastic vertical vein. This may be associated with asplenia or polysplenia.

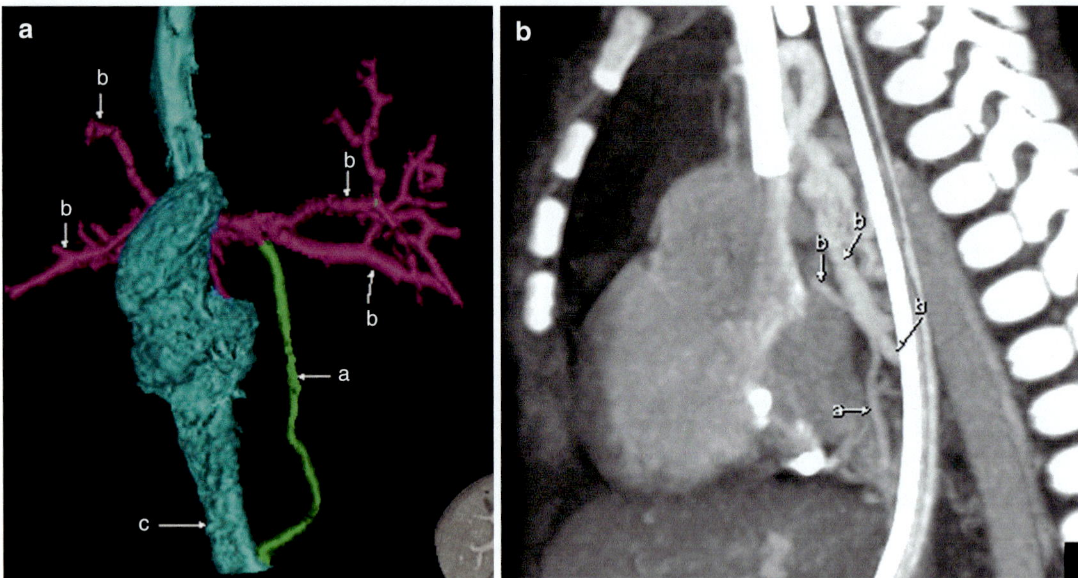

Fig. 5.10 Frontal oblique 3D color model (**a**) and sagittal MIP image (**b**) demonstrating multiple pulmonary veins (*b*) draining to a markedly hypoplastic vertical vein (*a*), which connects to the IVC (*c*)

Mixed-Type TAPVR

Mixed-type TAPVR, the least common form, is a combination of the previously described anomalous connections. In this condition, CTA is effective in delineating complex anatomy.

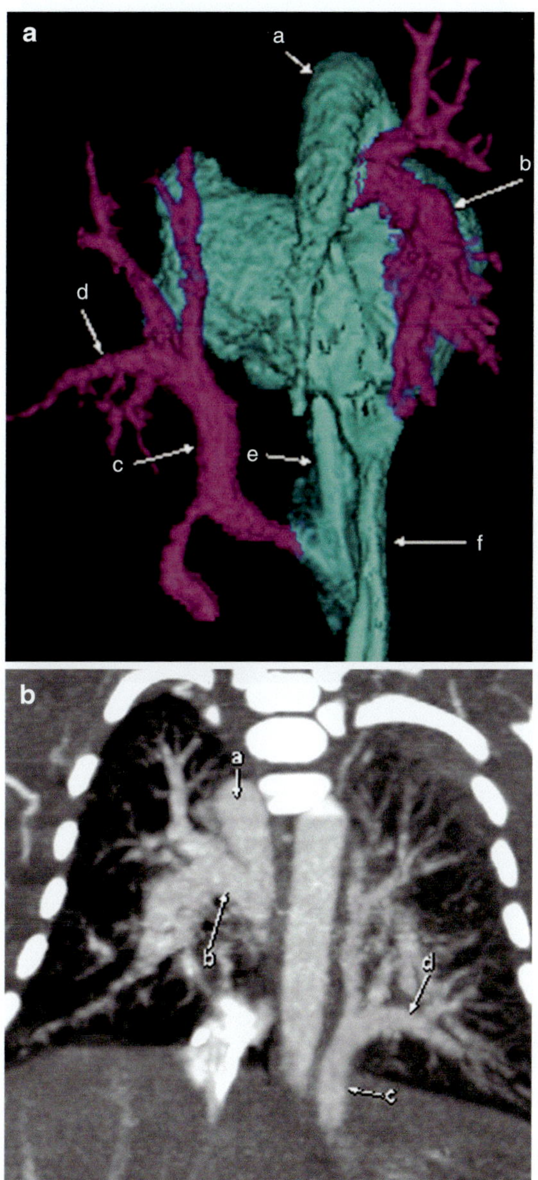

Fig. 5.11 Posterior projection of a 3D color model (**a**) and coronal MIP image (**b**) demonstrating mixed-type TAPVR. The left pulmonary veins (*d*) drain to the IVC (*e* and *f*) via a vertical vein (*c*). The right pulmonary veins (*b*) drain directly to the azygous vein (*a*)

Hypogenetic Lung (Scimitar) Syndrome

In hypogenetic lung syndrome, also known as scimitar syndrome, there is a triad of findings: (1) PAPVR of the right lung, typically to the IVC or right atrium, (2) a hypoplastic right lung and right pulmonary artery, and (3) a systemic arterial supply to the right lower lobe. Patients are acyanotic and typically asymptomatic. The name *scimitar* comes from the curved appearance of the right lower lobe pulmonary vein, which becomes larger as it approaches the diaphragm and may look like a scimitar sword, especially on chest radiography.

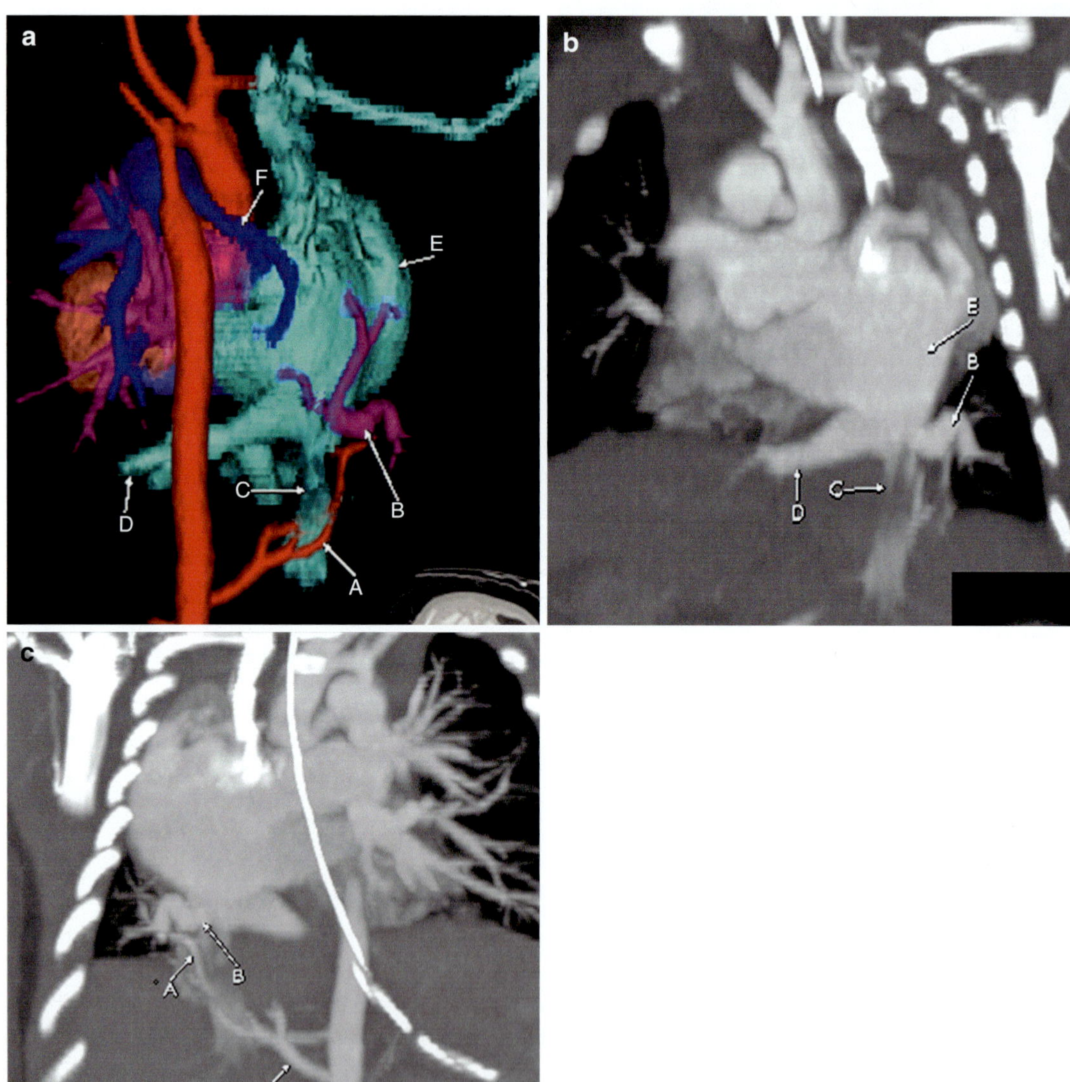

Fig. 5.12 Posterior projection color-coded 3D model (**a**) and coronal MIP images (**b** and **c**) from a chest CTA showing right lower lobe partial anomalous venous return (*B*) to the junction between the IVC (*C*) and right atrium (*E*). There also is a systemic arterial supply (*A*) to the right lower lobe from the descending aorta and a hypoplastic right pulmonary artery (*F*). Notice the drainage of the hepatic veins (*D*) to the right atrium

Azygous Continuation of the IVC

In azygous continuation, the prehepatic suprarenal IVC is interrupted, with most of the lower extremity venous return occurring through a dilated azygos (usually) or hemiazygos vein; the intrahepatic IVC is absent. Typically, the hepatic veins form a confluence of a posthepatic IVC that drains normally into the right atrium. Rarely, the hepatic veins drain directly into the right atrium. This condition is associated with ASD, ventricular septal defect (VSD).

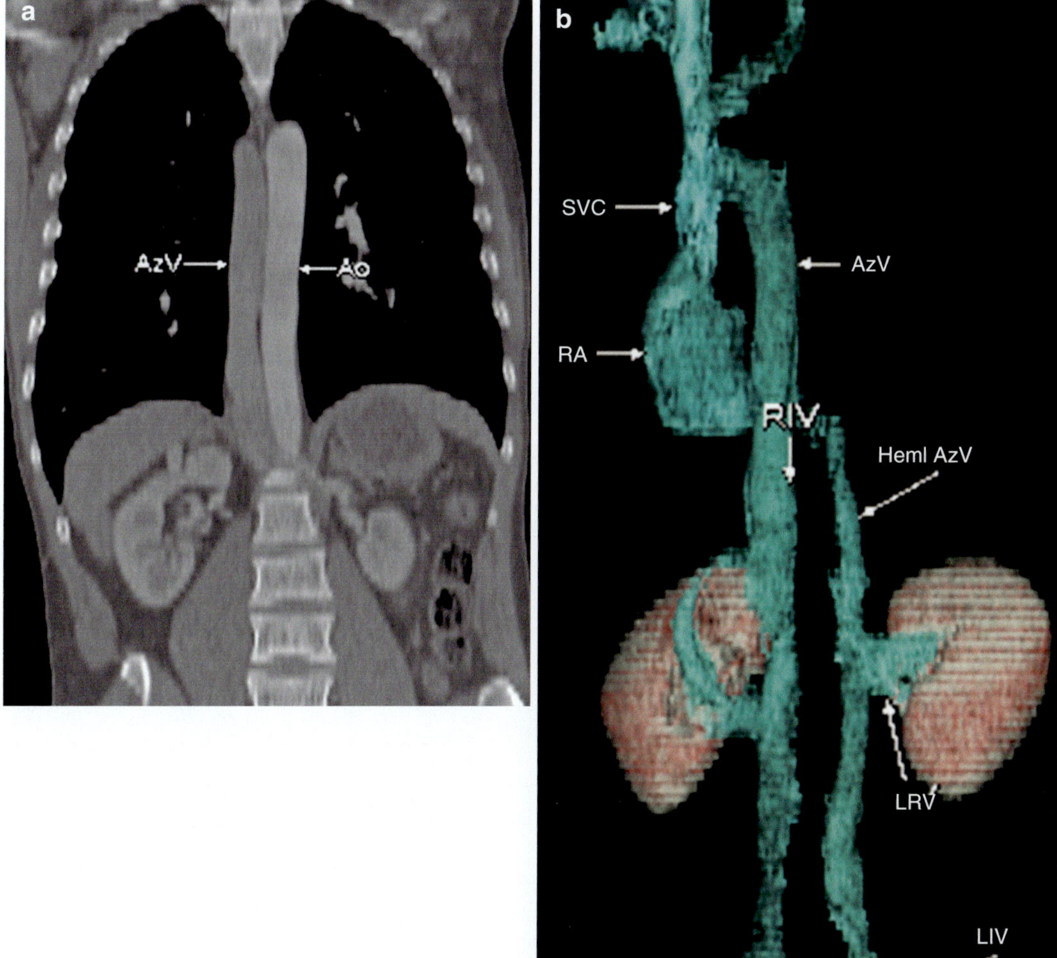

Fig. 5.13 Coronal MIP image (**a**) and anterior projection of a 3D color model (**b**) demonstrating a markedly dilated azygos vein (*AzV*) receiving inflow from an interrupted IVC (*RIV*) and the hemiazygos vein (*Hemi AzV*). Left-sided lower-extremity blood drains to the left common iliac vein (*LIV*), which coalesces with the left renal vein (*LRV*) into the Hemi AzV (variant duplicated caval system). No intrahepatic IVC was present on subsequent images. *Ao* aorta, *SVC* superior vena cava, *RA* right atrium

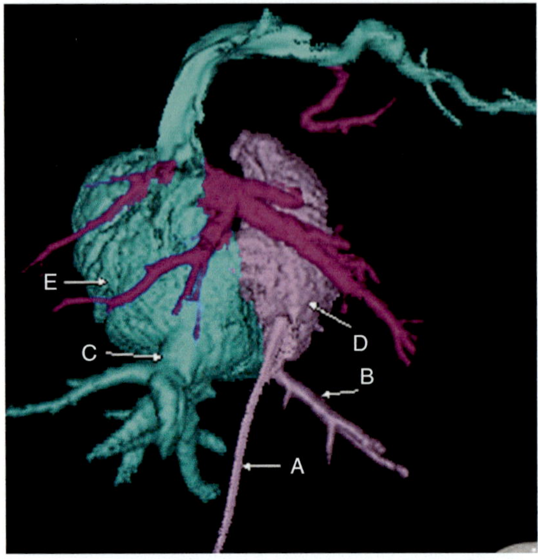

Fig. 5.14 Posterior projection of a 3D color CTA scan showing an umbilical venous catheter (*A*) coursing through one of the right-sided hepatic veins (*B*) to enter the right aspect of the right atrium (*D*). A left-sided IVC (*C*) enters the left aspect of the right atrium (*E*) as well. The presence of normal anatomic hepatic venous drainage in addition to a left IVC is evidence of a duplicated caval system

Duplicated (Bilateral) IVC

In duplicated, or bilateral, IVC, the left common iliac vein ascends to the left of the aorta rather than merging with the right common iliac vein. At the level of the left renal vein, it receives renal inflow and usually crosses anterior to the aorta to unite with the right-sided IVC. Duplicated IVC may be asymmetric, with the right side usually dominant and larger. Incomplete IVC duplication is common (see Fig. 5.13), with only separation of the hepatic venous drainage.

Patent Foramen Ovale

In patent foramen ovale (PFO), there is a normal interatrial channel in the posteroinferior atrial septum that allows blood flow to bypass the pulmonary circulation *in utero*. At birth, because the left atrial pressure exceeds the pressure in the right atrium, a preexisting left atrial tissue flap closes the channel across the fossa ovalis. This usually is permanent. It may remain open in conditions in which the right atrial pressure is elevated, such as tricuspid atresia or Ebstein's anomaly. An asymptomatic right-to-left shunt may exist into adulthood.

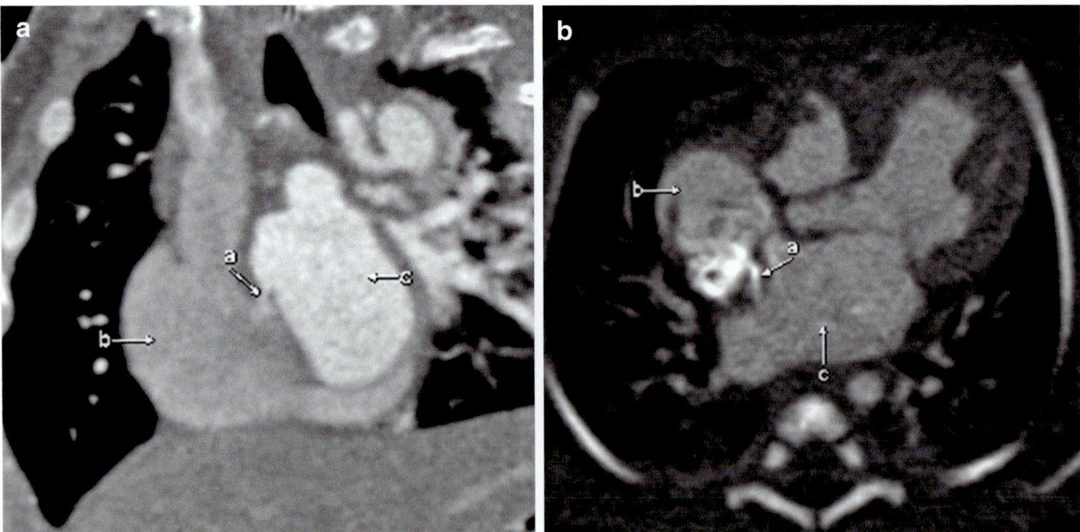

Fig. 5.15 Coronal (**a**) and axial MIP (**b**) images demonstrating a jet of contrast passing through a PFO (*a*) between the right (*b*) and left (*c*) atria

Ostium Secundum ASD

Ostium secundum ASD is the most common ASD type. It is located in the midportion of the atrial septum and typically is a result of the deficiency of the atrial septum primum to form a flap with the atrial septum secundum. It may be asymptomatic into adulthood or eventually result in shunt reversal and Eisenmenger's syndrome. It may close spontaneously or require percutaneous intervention and flap closure.

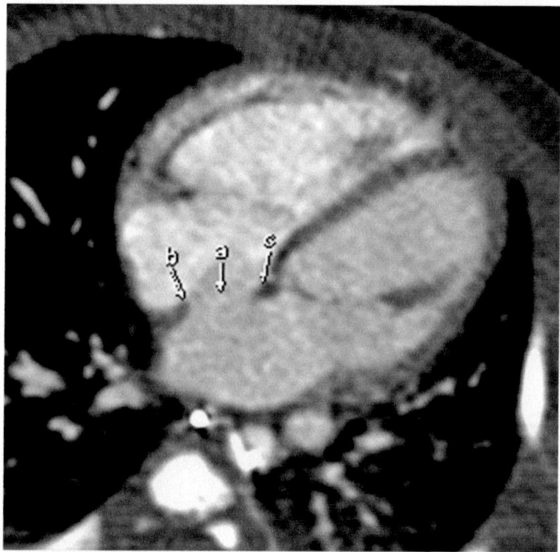

Fig. 5.16 Axial image showing a large secundum-type ASD (*a*) bordered by the posteromedial (*b*) and anterolateral (*c*) flaps of the atrial septum

Ostium Primum ASD

In ostium primum ASD, the most basic of the endocardial cushion/AV septal defects, the most anteroinferior atrial septum is deficient. This condition may coexist with a defect in the anterior mitral valve leaflet and may or may not be associated with a VSD.

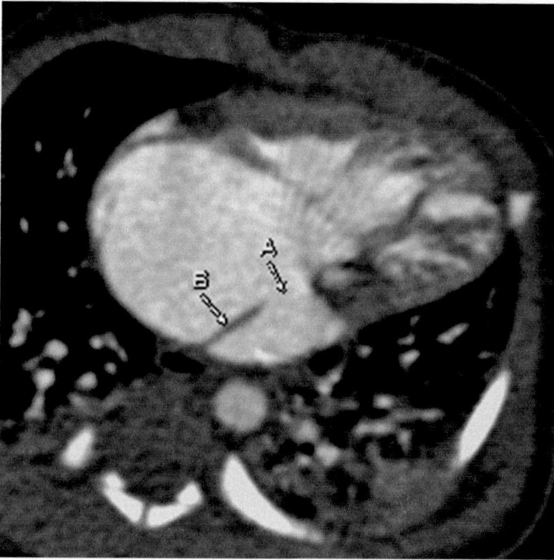

Fig. 5.17 Axial CTA image demonstrating an interatrial connection through a septum primum–type ASD (*A*). The posterior atrial septum (*B*) is intact

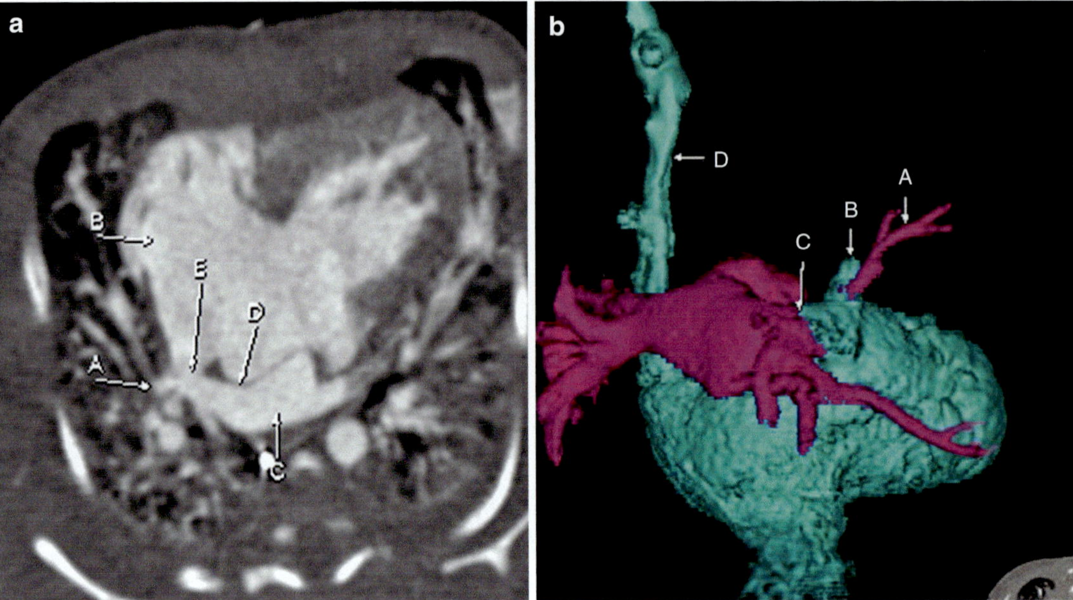

Fig. 5.18 Axial cardiac CTA (**a**) and posterior projection 3D model (**b**) images showing a posterosuperior defect (*E*) in the atrial septum (*D*) with communication between the left (*C*) and right atria (*B* in axial image). This nearly always is associated with PAPVR of the right upper lobe (*A*), which drains to the junction of the SVC (*B* in 3d image) and right atrium

Sinus Venosus–Type ASD

Sinus venosus–type ASD occurs in the posterosuperior or posteroinferior atrial septum and is contiguous with the SVC or IVC, respectively. It nearly always is associated with right upper lobe PAPVR because of the deficiency of the septum separating the right atrium from the left atrial–right pulmonary venous junction. Occasionally, a pulmonary vein is inserted high up the SVC, distant from the sinus venosus ASD.

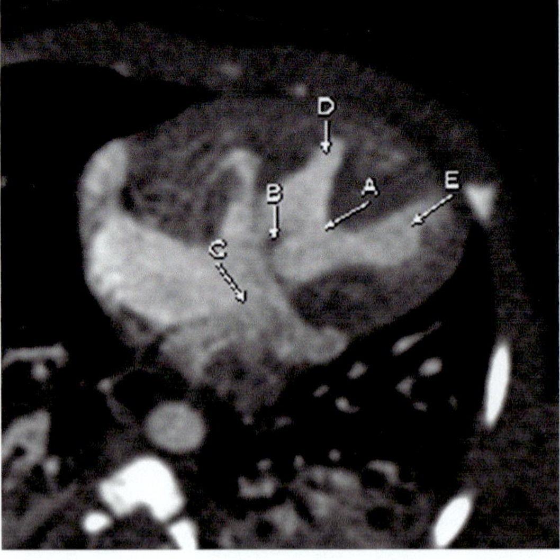

Fig. 5.19 Axial CTA image demonstrating a septum primum ASD (*C*) as well as a posterior-type VSD (*A*). Blood from the atria and from the left (*E*) and right (*D*) ventricles may mix freely. A common AV valve (*B*) is present.

Complete AV Septal Defect (Complete Common AV Canal Defect)

Complete AV septal defect is a defect in the development of the endocardial cushion to form the tricuspid and mitral valves, and to complete the septation of the atrial septum and ventricular septum. This results in a common AV valve with variable chordal attachments to the ventricle, ostium primum ASD, and AV canal–type (inlet) VSD. This may be associated with trisomy 21 as well as heterotaxy syndromes. There also may be a concomitant presence of tetralogy of Fallot.

Tricuspid Atresia

Tricuspid atresia is a congenital agenesis of the right AV (tricuspid) valve, preventing forward flow of systemic venous blood from the right atrium to the ventricle. Newborns with tricuspid atresia must have a coexisting ASD to survive. This condition may be associated with a VSD allowing pulmonary perfusion, or transposition of the great arteries. The size of the heart depends on the size of the VSD. If there is no VSD and the great arteries have a normal relationship, there will be pulmonary atresia, and the patient requires ductal patency for survival.

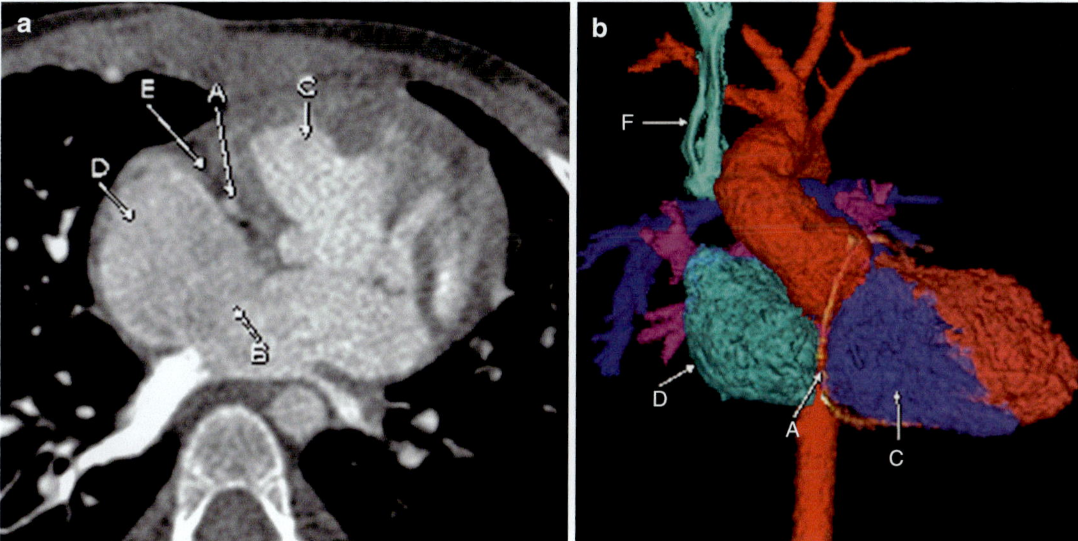

Fig. 5.20 (**a**) Axial CTA image showing fat (*E*) and fibrous tissue, with the right coronary artery (*A*) in the expected location of the tricuspid valve. Blood cannot pass directly from the right atrium (*D*) to the right ventricle (*C*), so it crosses through an ASD (*B*) into the left atrium. (**b**) Anterior projection 3D model demonstrating SVC (*F*) drainage to the pulmonary arteries from a post-surgical Glenn shunt

Ebstein's Anomaly

In Ebstein's anomaly, the septal leaflets of the tricuspid valve may be dysplastic, hypoplastic, and displaced. The anterior leaflet typically is large and sail-like; it may have tethering into the RV free wall and may extend up to the RV outflow tract apically into the right ventricle, leading to "atrialization" of the right ventricle. The posterior variable degree of non-coaptation of the leaflets results in tricuspid regurgitation, which often is severe and results in massive cardiomegaly.

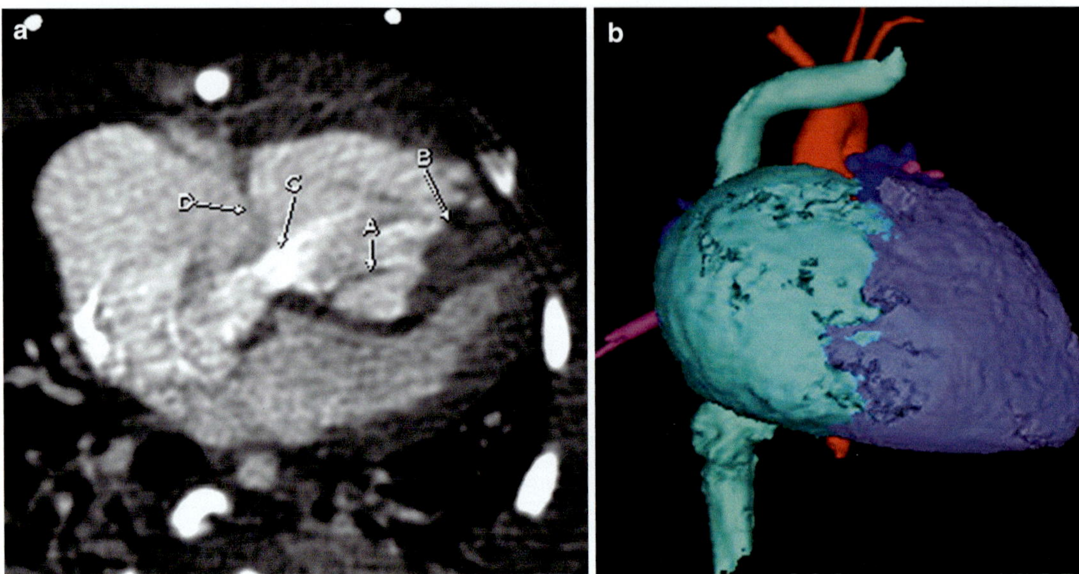

Fig. 5.21 (**a**) Axial cardiac CTA image demonstrating the sail-like, apically displaced septal leaflet (*A*) of the tricuspid valve, which is tented by dysplastic cordae tendineae (*B*) seen along the apicoseptal portion of the left ventricle. The anterior leaflet (*D*) of the tricuspid valve is visualized in a relatively normal position. This causes regurgitation along the septal portion of the valve (*C*). (**b**) Frontal projection color 3D image showing massive dilatation of the right atrium (*light blue*) and right ventricle (*purple*)

Mitral Stenosis

Mitral stenosis may result from congenital heart disease or acquired heart disease, classically from rheumatic fever. In this condition, an impediment to left ventricular inflow results in left atrial enlargement. Eventually, elevated left atrial and pulmonary pressures result in pulmonary edema and pulmonary hypertension.

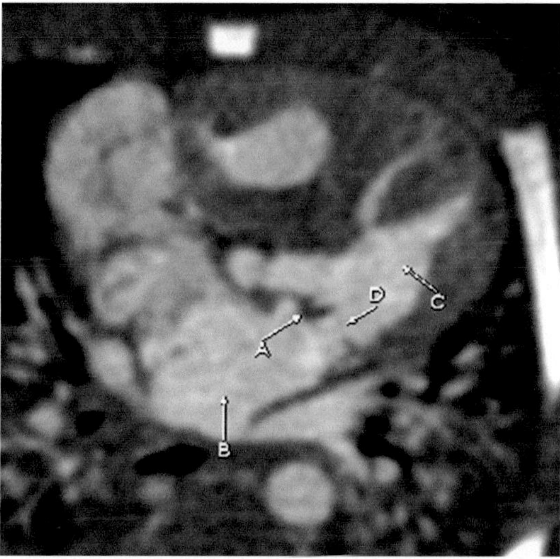

Fig. 5.22 Axial cardiac CTA image demonstrating a thickened anterior mitral leaflet (*A*), resulting in a stenotic mitral orifice (*D*) for oxygenated blood to flow from the left atrium (*B*) to the ventricle (*C*) during diastole. The left atrium is mildly enlarged

Single Atrium

Single atrium is the result of a development failure in the components of the atrial septum. This condition typically is part of a heterotaxy syndrome, usually with a complete AV septal leaflet. It may be associated with single ventricle, usually a single right ventricle.

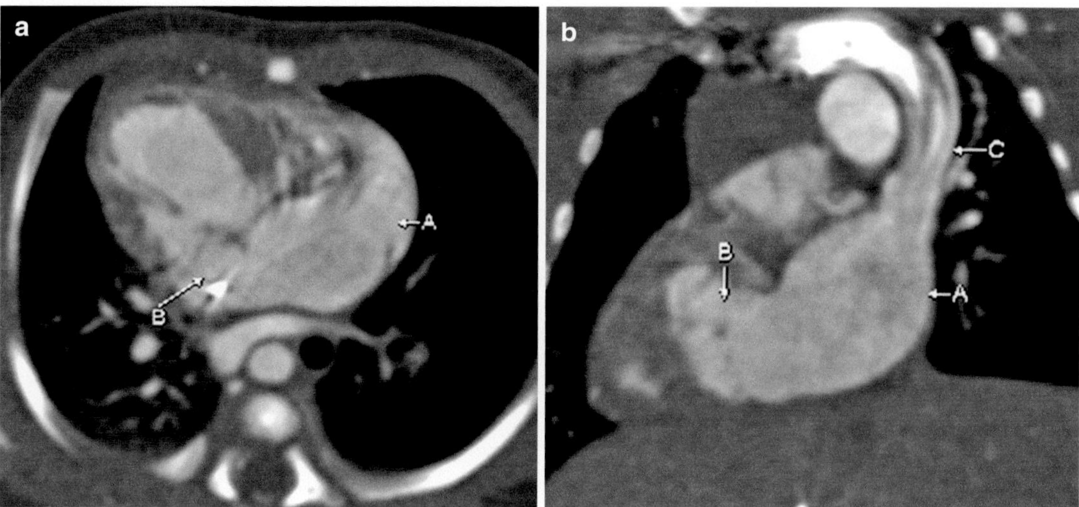

Fig. 5.23 Axial (**a**) and coronal (**b**) cardiac CTA images showing a right (*B*) and left (*A*) atria with no formed interatrial septum. Notice the left- sided SVC (*C*), which drains to the left atrium in this patient with asplenia-type heterotaxy

6 Evaluation of the Ventricles

Randy Ray Richardson and Taruna Ralhan

Evaluation of the ventricles comprises the following steps:

1. Distinguish the morphologic right ventricle from the left ventricle. The right ventricle typically has a more trabeculated septal surface than the left ventricle. The right ventricle has a more pyramidal shape, with a moderator band at its apex. The left ventricle has an ellipsoid shape and a smoother septal surface. The right ventricular outflow tract (RVOT) or infundibulum is muscle bound and typically not in fibrous continuity with the tricuspid valve.
2. Look for ventricular septal defects (VSDs). These are seen most commonly in the perimembranous region of the ventricular septum but also may be observed in the muscular portion of the septum, subvalvular region, or posteriorly along the septum in patients with atrioventricular (AV) septal defects.
3. Evaluate ventricular size, motion, and function if sufficient data are available.
4. Look for an abnormally thickened myocardium, which may be a primary or secondary abnormality and may lead to outflow tract obstruction.

R.R. Richardson, MD (✉)
Department of Radiology,
St. Joseph's Hospital and Medical Center,
Creighton University School of Medicine,
West Thomas Rd 350, 85013
Phoenix, AZ, USA
e-mail: randy.richardson2@chw.edu,
randy.richardson2@dignityhealth.org

T. Ralhan, MD
Radiology Residency Program,
St. Joseph's Hospital and Medical Center,
Phoenix, AZ, USA

VSDs

VSDs are seen most commonly in the perimembranous region of the ventricular septum but also may be observed in the muscular portion of the septum, subvalvular region, and posteriorly along the septum in patients with AV septal defects. Ventricular size, motion, and function should be evaluated when sufficient data are available. Abnormally thickened myocardium may be a primary or secondary abnormality and may lead to outflow tract obstruction. Identification of the right and left ventricles may be difficult. Typically, the right ventricle is more trabeculated than the left ventricle. A moderator band may help identify the right ventricle, which may be important in patients with transposition.

R.R. Richardson, *Atlas of Pediatric Cardiac CTA*,
DOI 10.1007/978-1-4614-0088-2_6, © Springer Science+Business Media New York 2013

Normal Anatomy

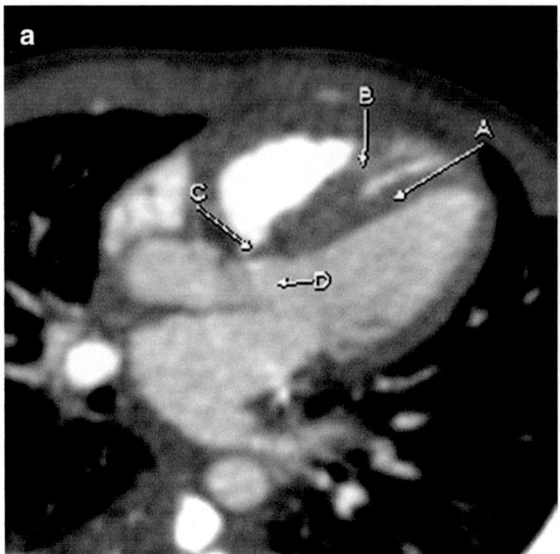

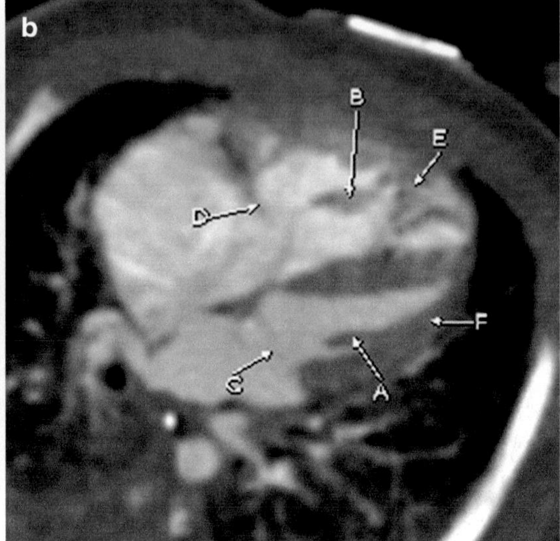

Fig. 6.1 (**a**, **b**) Two axial views from a cardiac CTA demonstrating the typical anatomy of the right and left ventricles. (**a**) A prominent moderator band (*B*), which extends from the interventricular septum (*A*) to the free wall of the right ventricle. Notice how thin the membranous portion of the interventricular septum is compared to the more muscular portion (*A*). The adjacent left ventricular outflow tract is shown (*D*). The left ventricular wall typically is smooth and compacted (*F*) with papillary muscles (*A*). (**b**) The right ventricle demonstrates trabeculations (*E*) cordae tendinae(*B*). The mitral valve (*C*) regulates blood flow from the left atrium to the left ventricle, and the tricuspid valve (*D*) regulates blood from the right atrium to the right ventricle

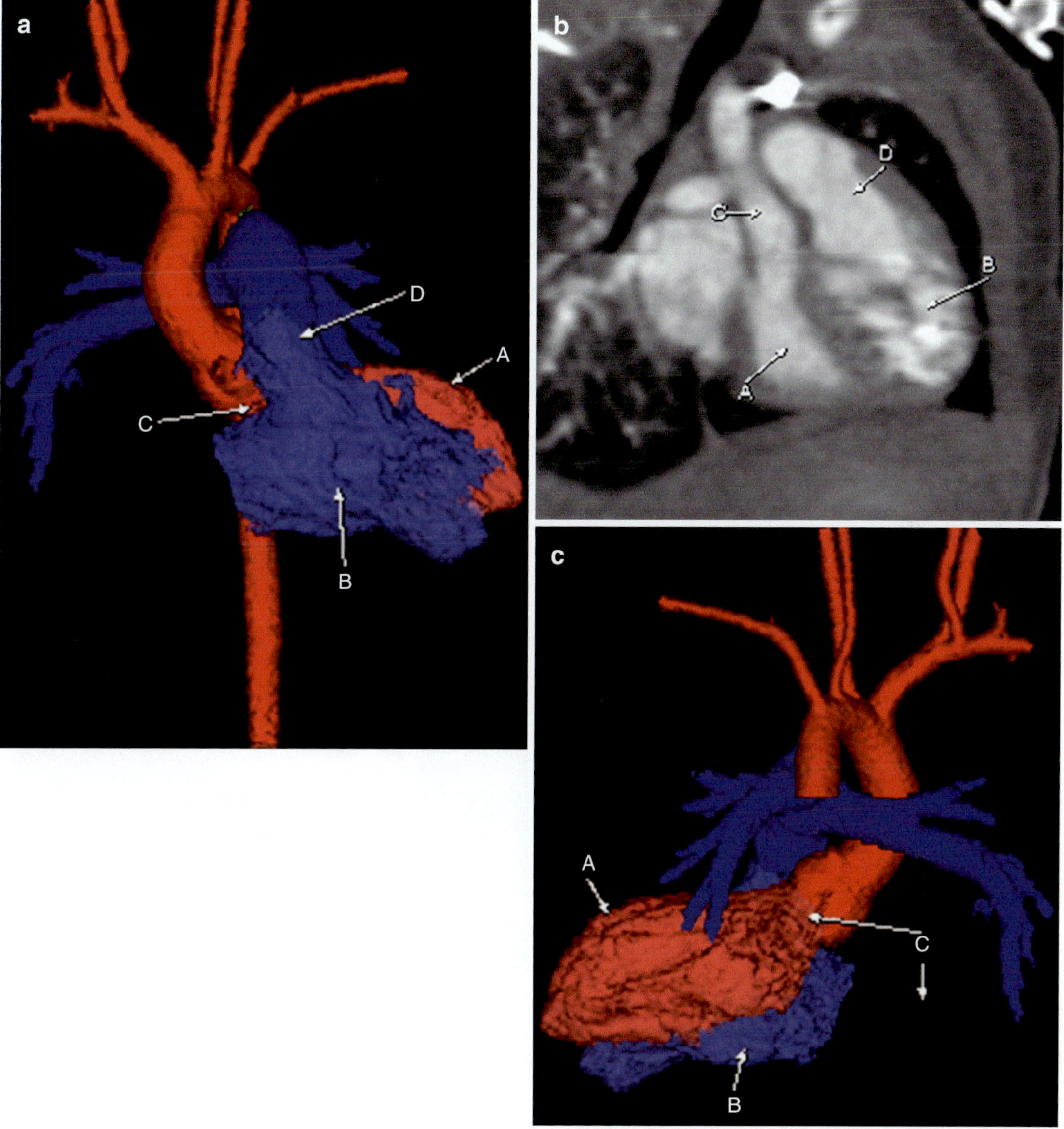

Fig. 6.2 Frontal (**a**) and posterior (**c**) projection color-coded three-dimensional (3D) images, as well as an oblique view of the ventricles and outflow tracts (**b**), demonstrating a normal RVOT (*D*) originating from the more trabeculated right ventricle (*B*). The RVOT (*D*) is anterior to and to the left of the left ventricular outflow tract (LVOT; *C*). The LVOT arises from the more conically shaped left ventricle (*A*)

Membranous-Type VSD

Membranous-type VSD is also called *perimembranous septal defect* because the membranous septum is very small and the defect usually extends to the muscular septum. A membranous VSD is the most common type, accounting for 75–80 % of all VSDs. The defect lies in the outflow tract of the left ventricle immediately below the aortic valve. Tachypnea generally is the initial presenting symptom. Clinical symptoms depend on the size of the VSD. Small defects cause heart murmur with no other clinical symptoms. Moderate to large VSDs may cause tachycardia, diaphoresis, and failure to thrive. Congestive heart failure eventually may occur.

Echocardiography is the main diagnostic modality. In patients with large defects, chest radiography may show cardiomegaly with increased pulmonary vascularity. Kerley B lines from interstitial pulmonary edema may be seen in some cases. The location of the VSD is important for surgical repair.

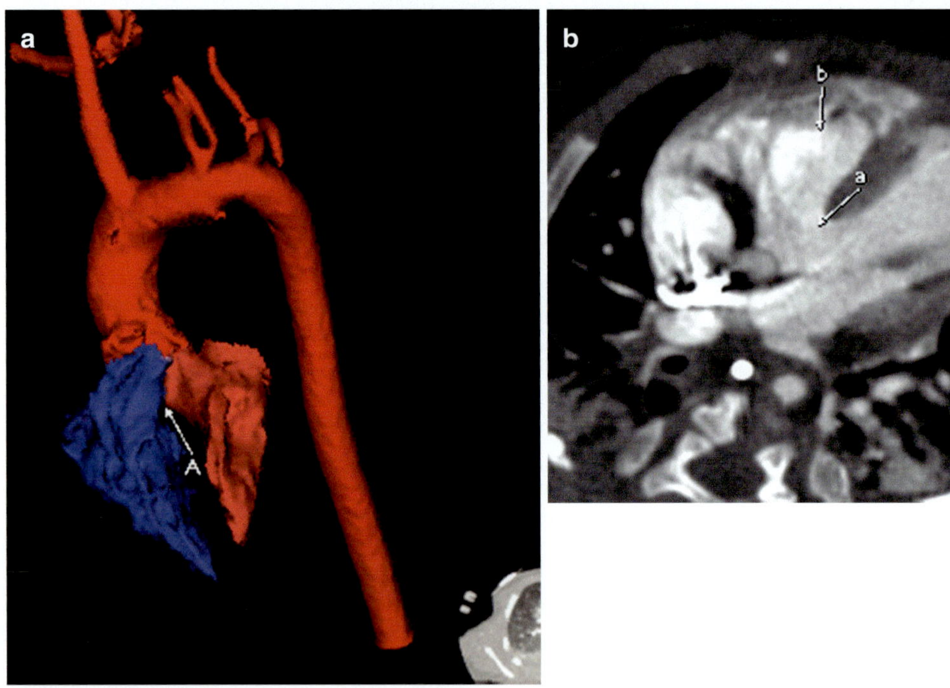

Fig. 6.3 Color-coded 3D reconstruction (**a**) and contrast-enhanced axial cardiac CT image (**b**). A large perimembranous VSD (*A*) between the right (*blue*) and left (*salmon*) ventricles is demonstrated on the 3D reconstruction images. Note that the defect lies immediately beneath the aortic valve. The axial cardiac CT image (**b**) demonstrates a large area of communication (*a*) between the left (*c*) and right (*b*) ventricles, consistent with a perimembranous VSD

Fig. 6.5 Color-coded 3D reconstruction (**a**) and contrast-enhanced axial cardiac CT image (**b**). Two areas of communication are seen (*a* and *b*) between the ventricles involving the muscular septum

Intramuscular-Type VSD

Intramuscular-type, or trabecular-type, VSD accounts for 5–20 % of all VSDs. The defect is bordered by muscle within the trabecular septum, away from the cardiac valves. These VSDs vary in size. Surgical treatment depends on the size of the defect. Small defects may close spontaneously during the first 2 years of life, most within the first 6 months.

Multiple Intramuscular VSDs

Multiple intramuscular VSDs may have a "Swiss cheese" appearance when obliquely oriented through the interventricular septum. Surgical management is complex, with increased morbidity and mortality compared with other types of VSD.

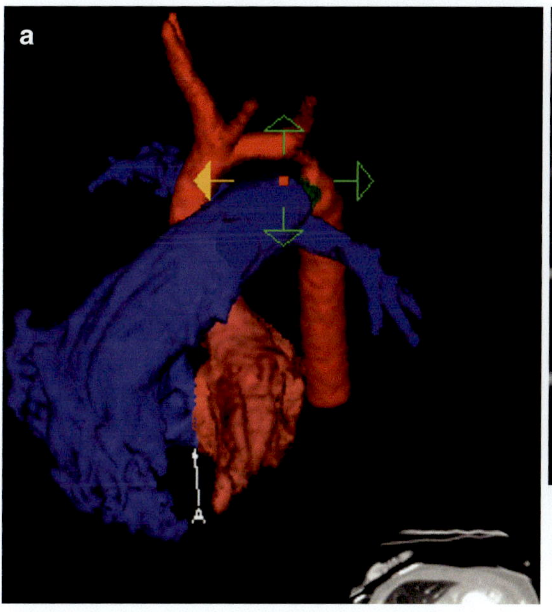

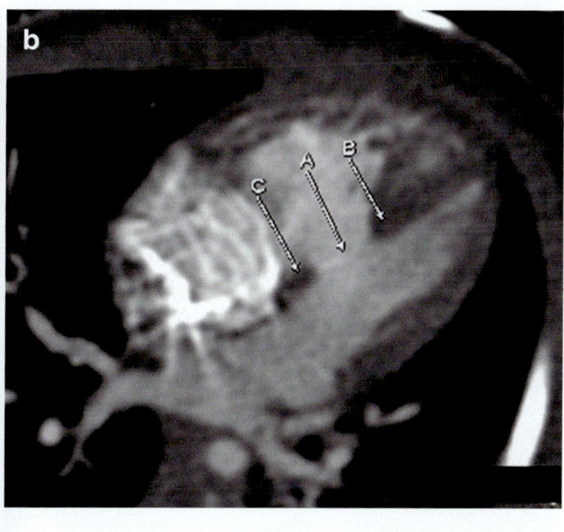

Fig. 6.4 Color-coded 3D reconstruction (**a**) and contrast-enhanced axial cardiac CT image (**b**). On the 3D reconstructed image, a VSD (*A*) is seen between the right (*purple*) and left (*pink*) ventricles. The corresponding axial CT image demonstrates the communication in the muscular interventricular septum (*A*). Notice that there is muscular tissue on the basilar (*C*) and apical (*B*) borders of the defect (*A*)

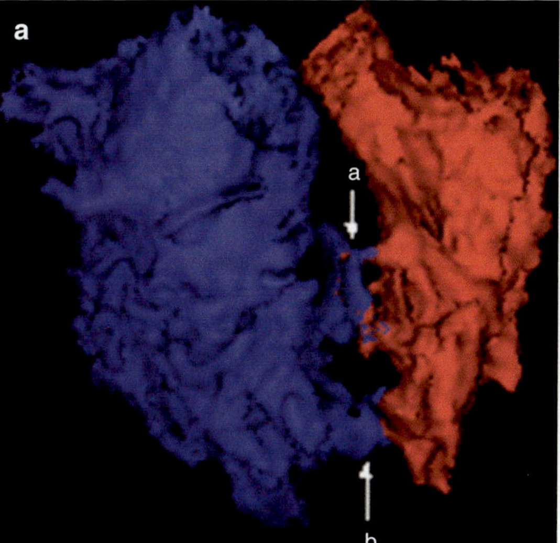

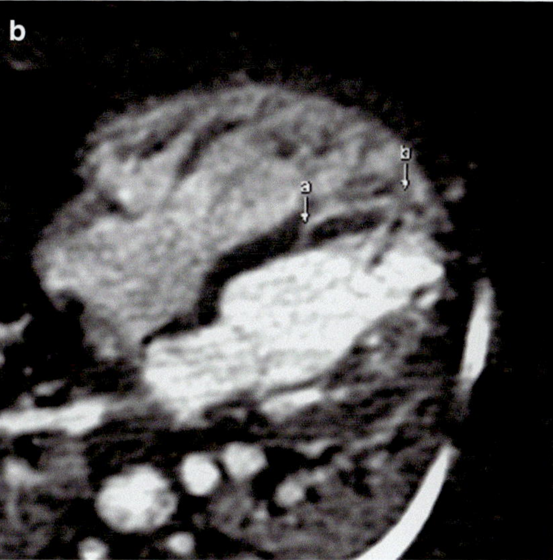

Posterior-Type VSD

Posterior-type, also known as AV septum– or inlet-type, VSD comprises 8–10 % of all VSDs. This defect, often associated with AV septal defect, occurs posterior to the septal leaflet of the tricuspid valve.

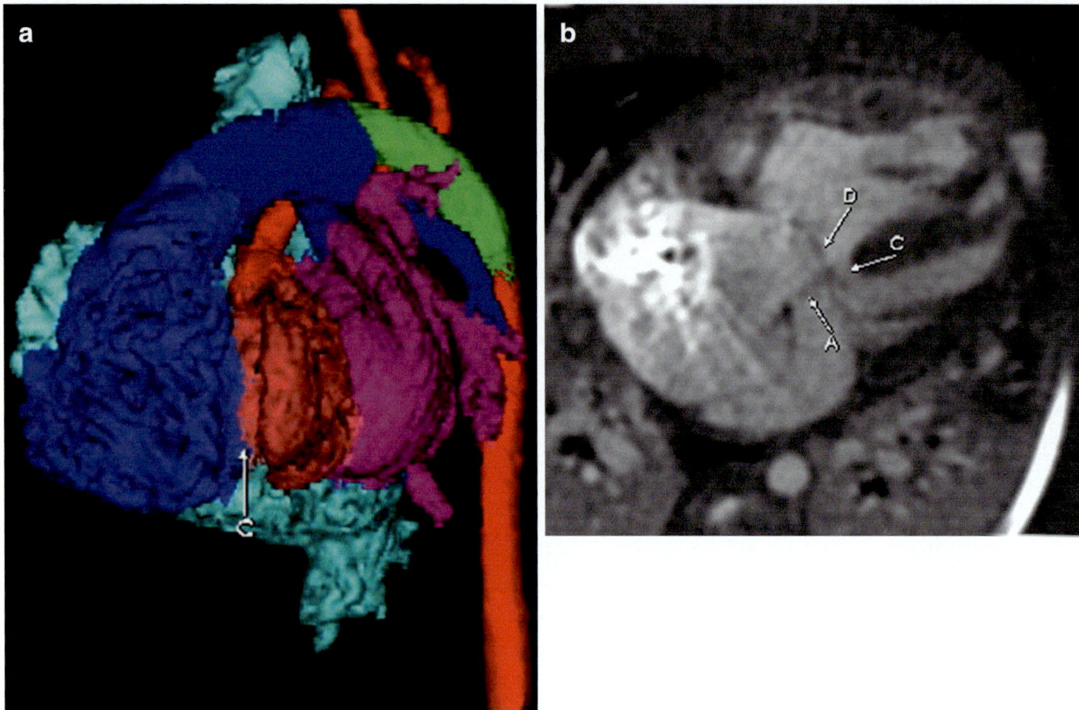

Fig. 6.6 Color-coded 3D reconstruction (**a**) and contrast-enhanced axial cardiac CT image (**b**). The 3D reconstructed image demonstrates abnormal communication between the ventricles posteriorly (*C*). The CT image demonstrates posterior-type VSD (*C*). Notice an associated septum primum defect (*A*) and a common AV valve (*D*). AV septal defects are associated with posterior-type VSD

Hypoplastic Left Heart Syndrome

Hypoplastic left heart syndrome is characterized by severe hypoplasia of the left ventricle and mitral valve and aortic atresia. It presents in the neonate with congestive heart failure and cyanosis. Patients with this condition depend on a patent ductus arteriosus (PDA).

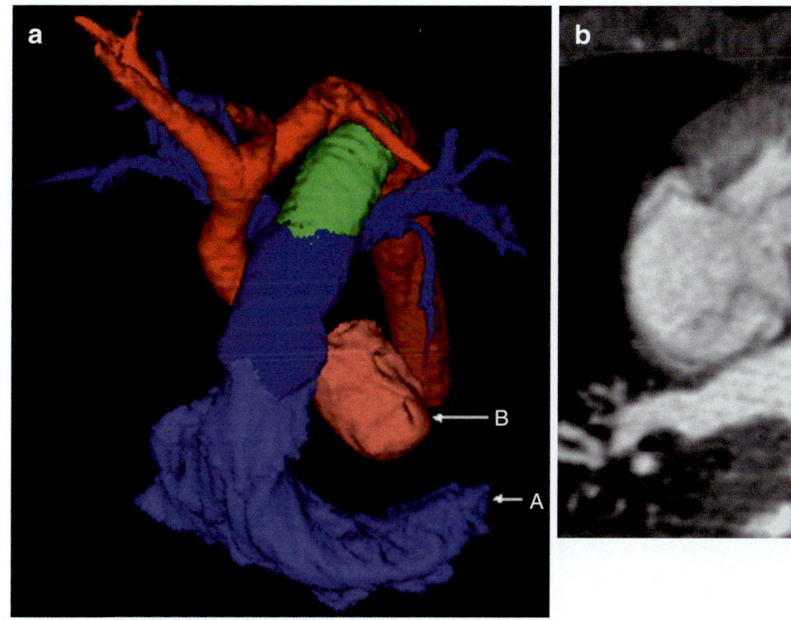

Fig. 6.7 Superior projection from a color-coded 3D image from a cardiac CTA (**a**) and axial image (**b**) demonstrating marked hypoplasia of the left ventricle (*B*). Notice how the right ventricle (*A*) wraps around the left ventricle (*B*). This finding is referred to as a *non–apex-forming left ventricle*

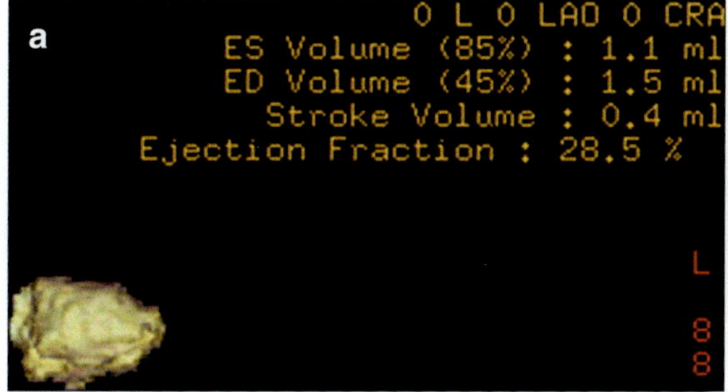

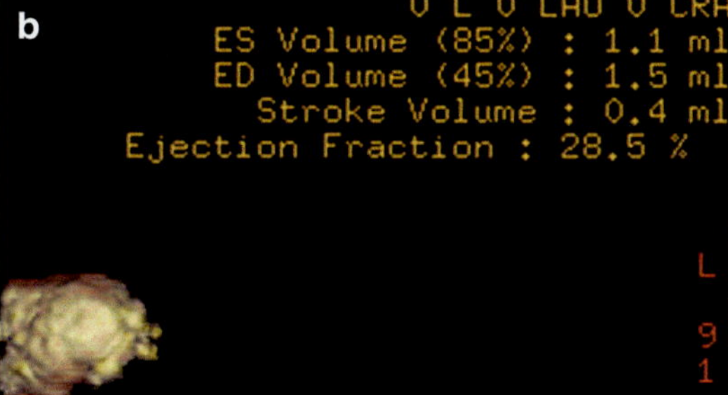

Fig. 6.8 Postprocessing of end-diastolic (**a**) and end-systolic (**b**) images from a patient with hypoplastic left heart syndrome. Function is poor, with a left ventricular ejection fraction of 28.5 %. Notice the dramatically small volumes in end systole and end diastole (1.1 and 1.5 mL). In the patient with a body surface area of 0.2, there was an end-systolic volume index of 5.5 mL/m^2 (normal, 17–37 mL/m^2) and an end-diastolic volume index of 7.5 mL/m^2 (normal, 50–84 mL/m^2).

Aortic Atresia/Hypoplastic Left Heart Syndrome

Aortic atresia is part of the hypoplastic left heart syndrome and involves hypoplasia/atresia of the ascending aorta, aortic valve, left ventricle, and mitral valve. Patients with this condition depend on a PDA for survival, with death occurring within days if it is untreated. Chest radiography demonstrates cardiomegaly and pulmonary venous congestion. Echocardiography, CT, MRI, and angiography may be used for treatment planning. A variety of surgical options exist, including the Norwood and hybrid procedures as well as heart transplantation in severe cases.

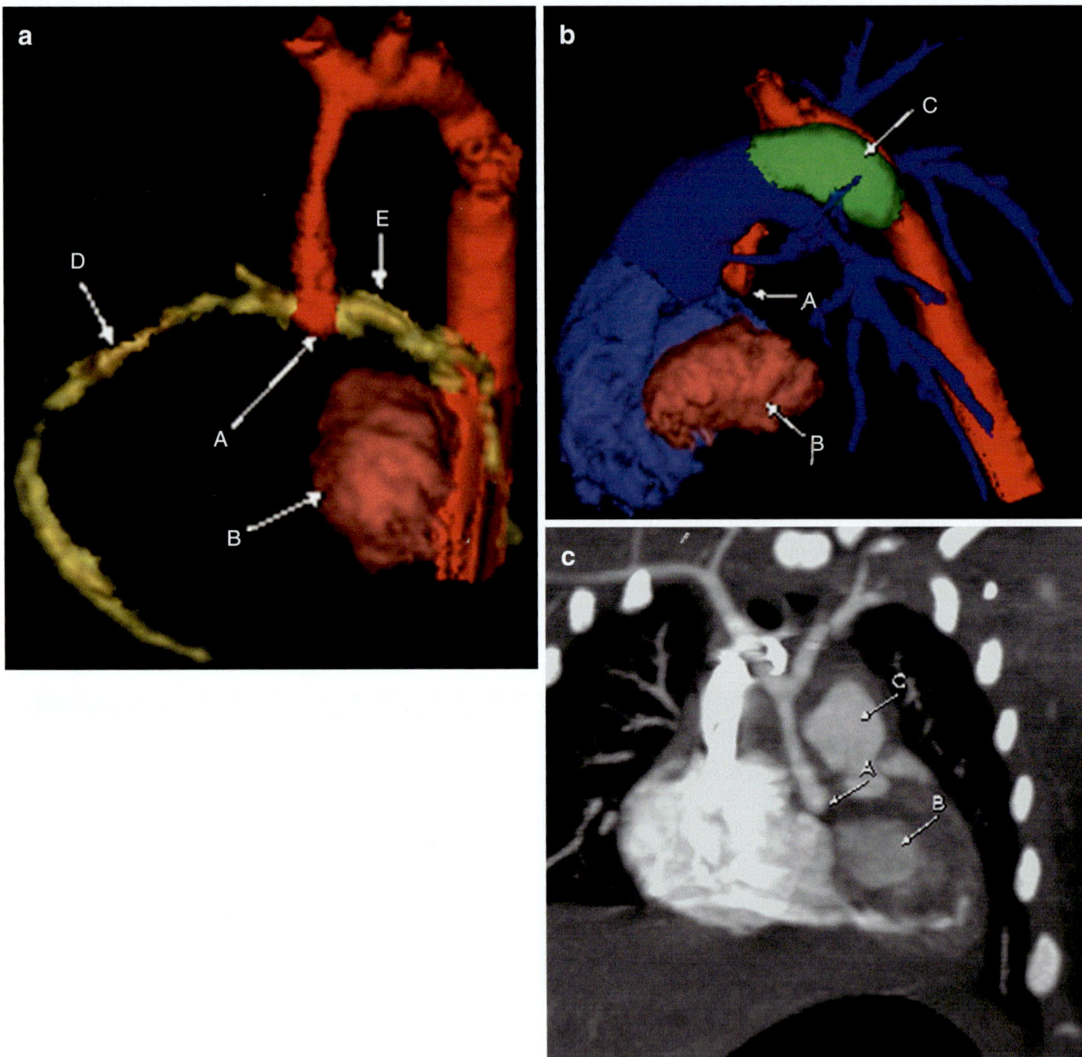

Fig. 6.9 Color-coded 3D (**a** and **b**) and coronal maximum-intensity projection (MIP; **c**) images from cardiac CT. The images demonstrate an atretic segment of the ascending aorta (*A*) at the aortic root, which is adjacent to a hypoplastic left ventricle (*B*). A large PDA is seen (*C*), which is necessary for short-term survival. Left (*E*) and right (*D*) coronary arteries are shown arising from the hypoplastic sinus of Valsalva of the proximal aorta

Hypoplastic Right Ventricle

Hypoplastic right heart syndrome is characterized by hypoplasia of the right ventricle, pulmonary valve, main pulmonary artery, and tricuspid valve. Hypoplastic right heart syndrome is less common than hypoplastic left heart syndrome. Coronary artery fistulas or coronary sinusoids often are present. Single-ventricle palliative procedures (Norwood) often are performed. Hypoplasia of the right ventricle often is seen in patients with pulmonic or tricuspid atresia. Flow to the lungs depends on a PDA. A non–apex-forming right ventricle is seen, with the left ventricle wrapping around the right.

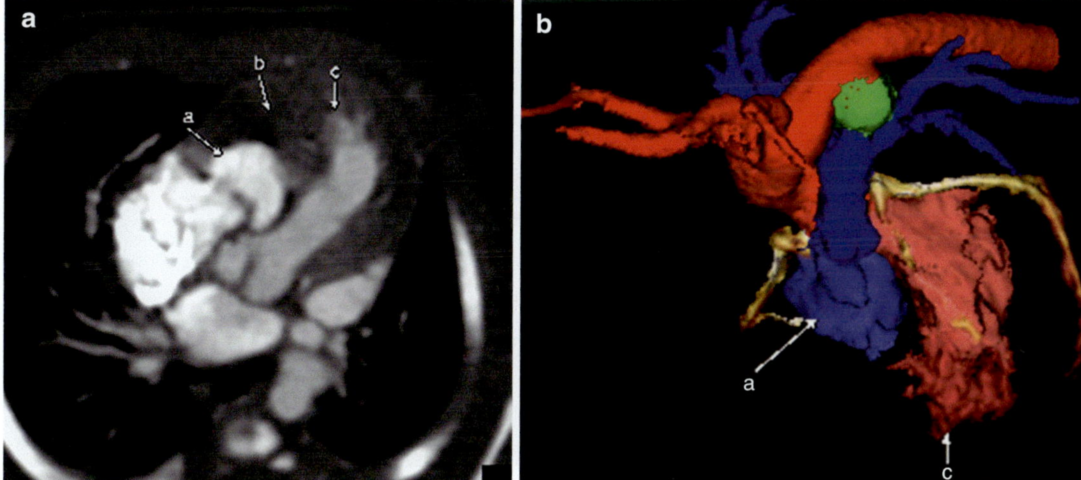

Fig. 6.10 Axial (**a**) and superior projection color-coded 3D (**b**) images from cardiac CTA showing marked right ventricular hypoplasia (*a*) with an apex-forming left ventricle (*c*) wrapping around the right ventricle (*a*), which is non–apex forming. Notice the very thick right ventricular wall (*b*) and the PDA (*green*)

Double-Inlet Left Ventricle

Double-inlet left ventricle is a condition in which both the right and left atria empty into the left ventricle. The right ventricle often is markedly hypoplastic (rudimentary) or absent, with essentially a common ventricle. Associated anomalies include transposition of the great vessels, pulmonic atresia, and pulmonic stenosis. The ventricles often are in a stacked or inverted position.

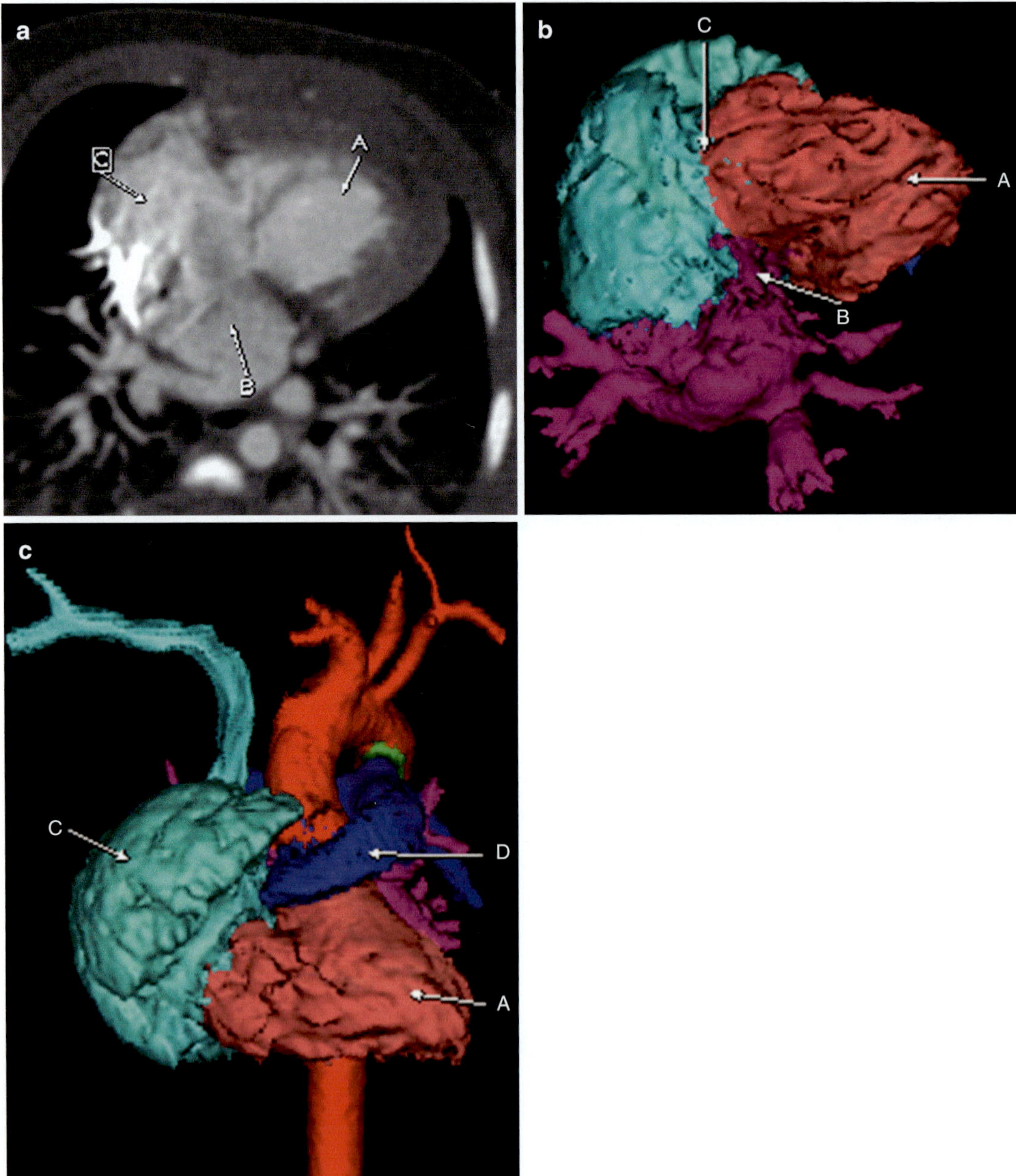

Fig. 6.11 Axial image (**a**) and inferior (**b**) and anterior (**c**) projections from a cardiac CTA. The right ventricle (*D*) is very hypoplastic (rudimentary); the left ventricle (*A*) is enlarged and receives blood from the right atrium (*C*) via the tricuspid valve and the left atrium (*B*) via the mitral valve. Notice the stacked appearance of the right (*D*) and left (*A*) ventricles with the right superior to the left

Single Ventricle

A single ventricle may be seen with a double-inlet left ventricle or may be seen with a common inlet to the ventricle with a common atrium. Other anomalies commonly seen with this defect include heterotaxy syndromes, transposition, and anomalies of venous return.

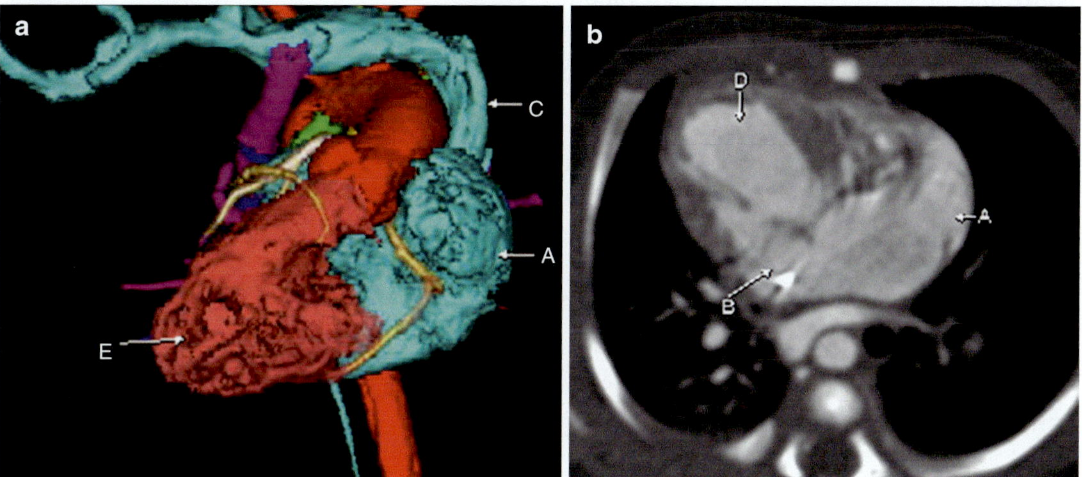

Fig. 6.12 Frontal projection color-coded (**a**) and axial cardiac CTA (**b**) images showing a single ventricle (*D* in **b**, *E* in **a**) with the absence of a pulmonary artery and pulmonary outflow tract. A common atrium also is present (*A*). Notice that there is situs inversus with the apex of the heart (*E*) on the right and the inferior vena cava (*C*) on the left. An anomalous vertical vein drains the pulmonary veins (*pink*). Notice that the umbilical venous catheter enters the right side of the common atrium (*B*)

Tetralogy of Fallot with Pulmonic Stenosis

Patients with tetralogy of Fallot (TOF) clasically have an overriding aorta, VSD (subaortic), RVOT stenosis or atresia, and right ventricular hypertrophy. TOF is a cyanotic heart disease with classic plain film x-ray findings of a normal heart size and decreased pulmonary vascularity. Right ventricular hypertrophy and a concave pulmonary artery segment give rise to the typical boot-shaped heart. Clinical severity depends on the degree of RVOT stenosis.

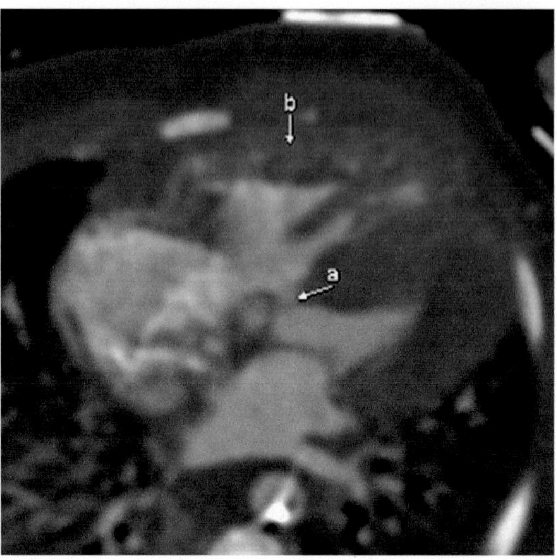

Fig. 6.13 Axial image from cardiac CT demonstrating thickening of the right ventricular wall (*b*) and a VSD (*a*) in a patient with TOF

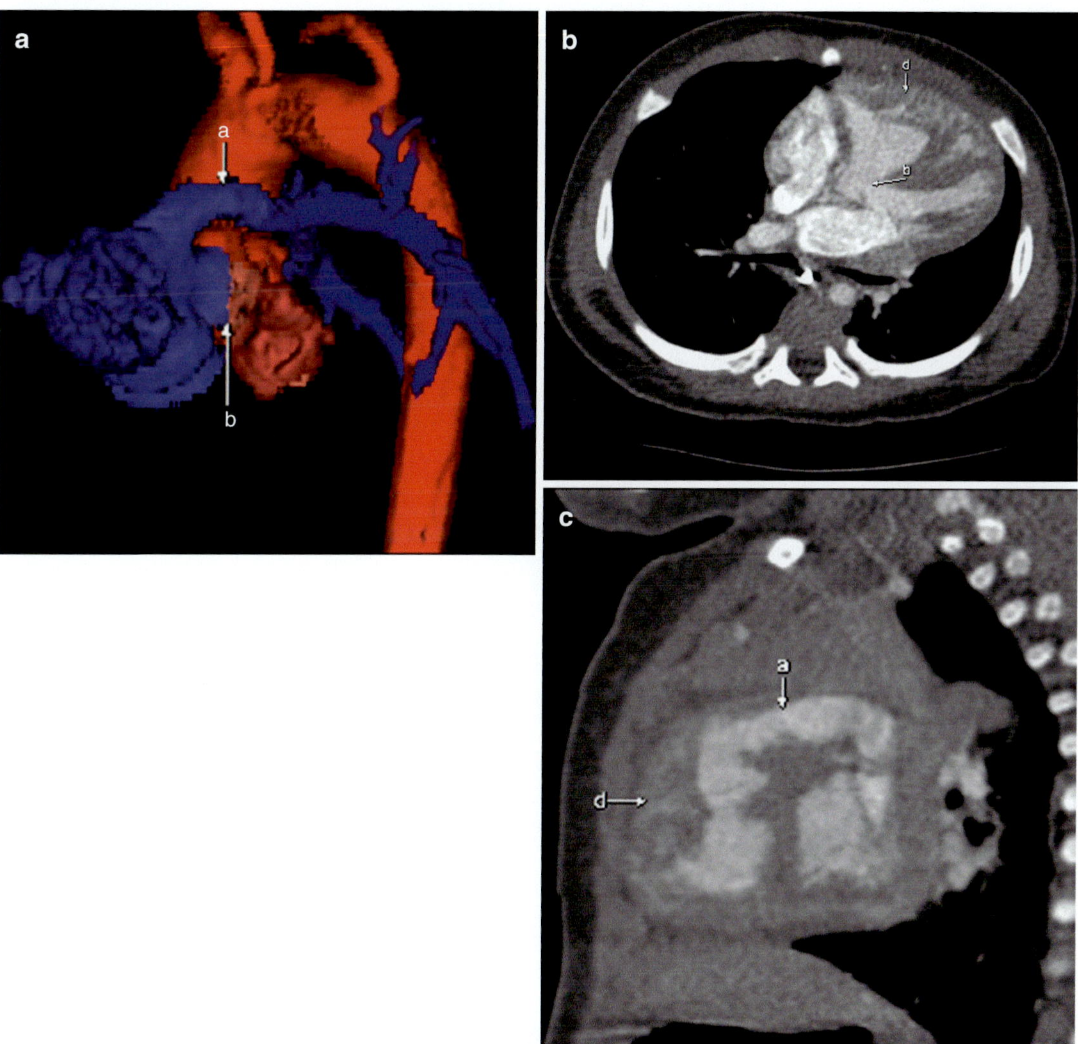

Fig. 6.14 Lateral projection 3D model (**a**) and axial and sagittal MIP images (**b** and **c**) from a cardiac CTA showing a narrowed infundibulum of the RVOT (*a*) with a VSD (*b*). Right ventricular hypertrophy (*d*) due to stenosis of the RVOT (*a*) is seen

TOF with PDA

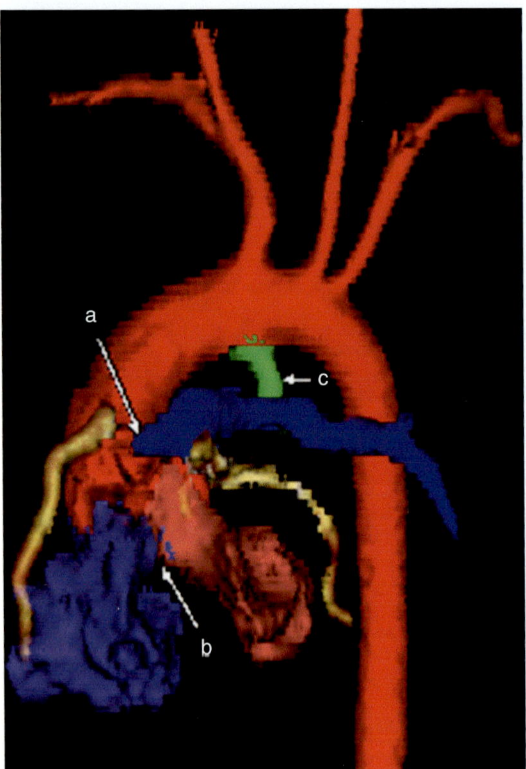

Fig. 6.15 Color-coded 3D image from a cardiac CTA showing pulmonic atresia (*a*) with a VSD (*b*) in a patient with TOF. Notice the PDA (*c*) extending from the undersurface of the aortic arch to the pulmonary arteries

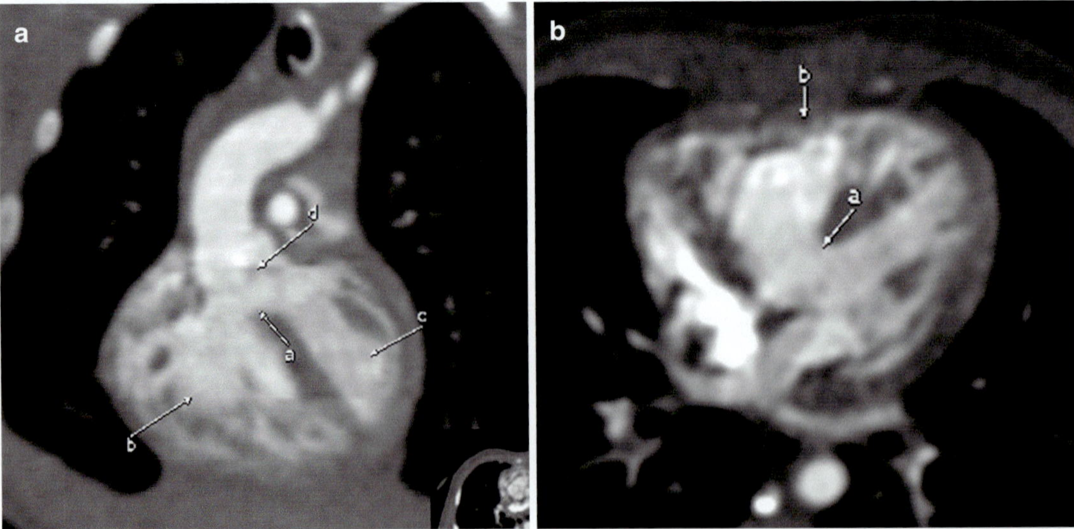

Fig. 6.16 Axial (**a**) and coronal (**b**) MIP images from cardiac CT showing a VSD (*a*) between the right (*b*) and left (*c*) ventricles with a typical overriding aorta (*d*). Notice how the aorta is positioned on top of the VSD (*a*) right between the right (*b*) and left (*c*) ventricles

TOF with Aortopulmonary Collaterals

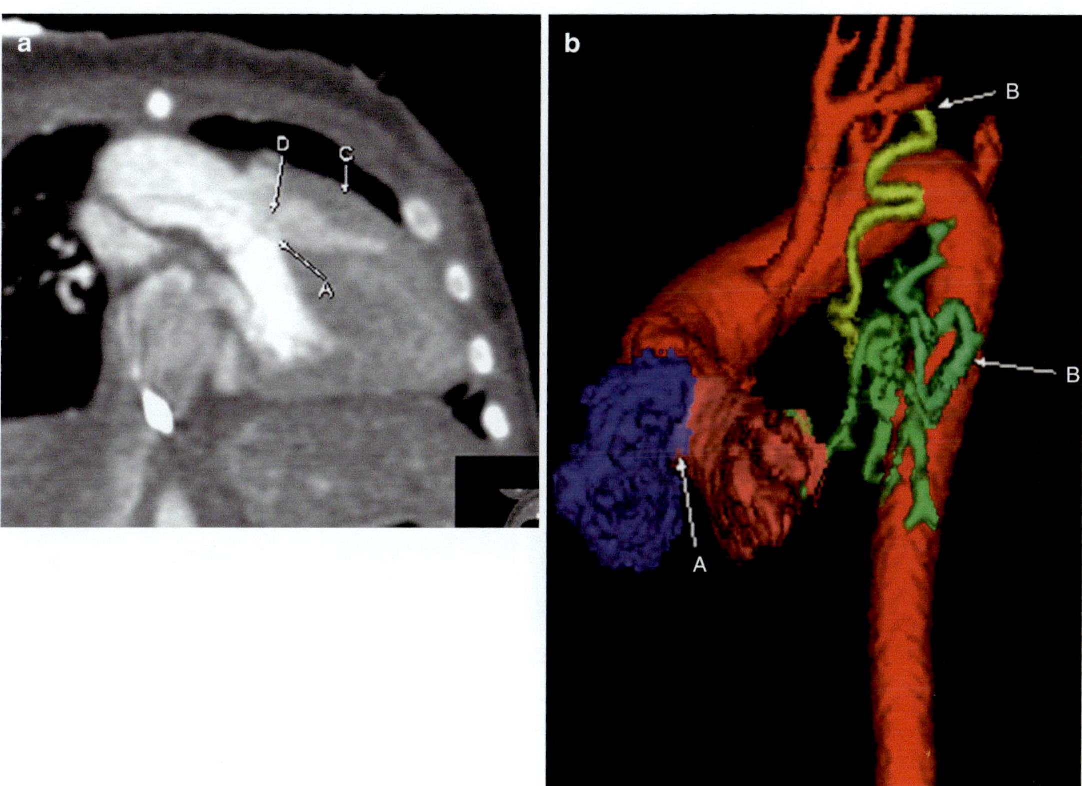

Fig. 6.17 Coronal MIP (**a**) and color-coded 3D (**b**) images demonstrating a VSD (*A*) with an overriding aorta (*D*) and thickening of the right ventricular wall (*C*). Aortopulmonary collaterals (*B*) provide circulation to the lungs in this patient with complete pulmonic atresia

TOF with Absence of the Pulmonic Valve

There is a variation of TOF in which the pulmonic valve is absent. There is moderate to severe pulmonic regurgitation through a stenotic RVOT with no pulmonary valve. The pulmonary arteries are markedly enlarged, frequently compressing the trachea and/or mainstem bronchi.

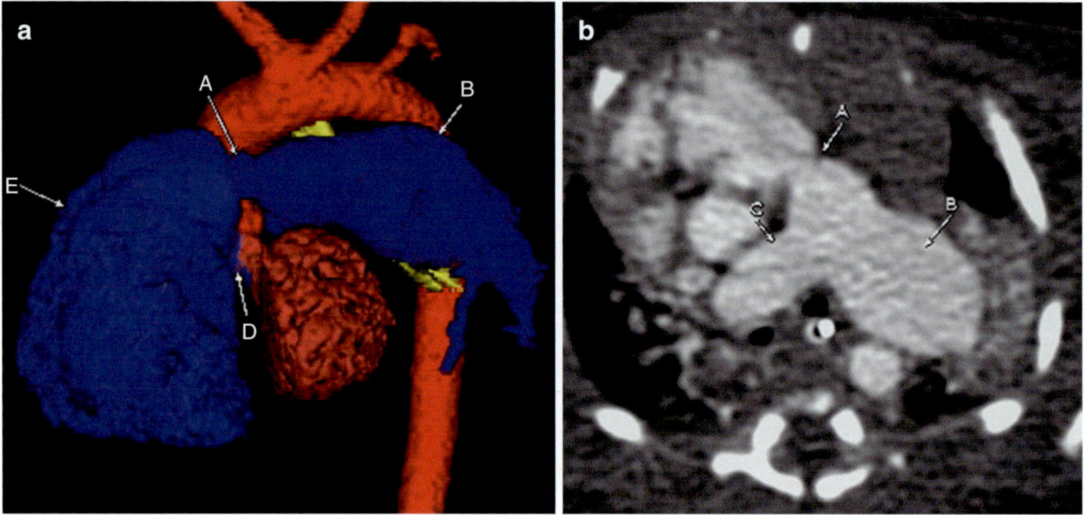

Fig. 6.18 Color-coded 3D (**a**) and axial MIP (**b**) images showing stenosis at the normal level of the pulmonic valve (*A*). With the absence of a pulmonic valve, there is dilatation of the right (*C*) and left (*B*) pulmonary arteries, along with dilatation of the right ventricle (*E*) due to severe pulmonic regurgitation. A VSD (*D*) also is demonstrated

7 Evaluation of the Great Vessels

Randy Ray Richardson and Travis Scharnweber

Evaluation of the great vessels should include the following:

(a) Outflow tracts. These may be switched, narrowed, absent, or aneurysmal.

(b) Aorta

  (i) It may be discontinuous (interruption of the aortic arch), stenotic in patients with coarctation of the aorta or supravalvular aortic stenosis, or hypoplastic.

  (ii) Identify whether the arch is on the left or right, and determine the number and location of vessels arising from the arch. Vascular rings, such as a double arch or right arch with an aberrant left subclavian artery, may cause airway obstruction.

  (iii) Look for aortopulmonary collaterals. These typically are seen along the descending aorta but may arise from the arch or great vessels.

  (iv) Measure the size and caliber of the aorta at the aortic annulus, sinus of Valsalva, sinotubular junction, transverse arch, and descending aorta. Comparison with normative data (z-score) may be helpful.

R.R. Richardson, MD (✉)
Department of Radiology,
St. Joseph's Hospital and Medical Center,
Creighton University School of Medicine,
West Thomas Rd 350, 85013 Phoenix, AZ, USA
e-mail: randy.richardson2@chw.edu,
randy.richardson2@dignityhealth.org

T. Scharnweber, MD
Radiology Residency Program,
St. Joseph's Hospital and Medical Center,
Phoenix, AZ, USA

(c) Pulmonary arteries

  (i) They may be atretic, hypoplastic, or anomalous. Determine the origin and course of the pulmonary arteries. Some pulmonary arteries may arise from the aorta, a patent ductus arteriosus (PDA), or the other pulmonary artery. (In pulmonary sling, the left pulmonary artery arises from the right and courses around the trachea, often causing tracheal or bronchial stenosis.)

  (ii) Evaluate the size of the main pulmonary artery and the right and left proximal and distal pulmonary arteries.

  (iii) Look for other vessels connected to the pulmonary arteries, such as a PDA. Aortopulmonary collaterals may be connected to the pulmonary arteries and may supply the lung directly.

(d) PDA

  (i) Typically, a PDA originates from the undersurface of the descending aorta or left brachiocephalic/subclavian artery but rarely may have other anomalous origins and may be bilateral, with one arising from the aorta and the other from the brachiocephalic artery.

  (ii) It may be large and tortuous, especially in patients with complex congenital heart disease. A diverticulum may be seen at the origin of the ductus (Kommerell's diverticulum). Look for mass effect from the enlarged PDA on other adjacent structures (especially the trachea and bronchi).

R.R. Richardson, *Atlas of Pediatric Cardiac CTA*,
DOI 10.1007/978-1-4614-0088-2_7, © Springer Science+Business Media New York 2013

(iii) Later in life, a calcification often is seen in the region of the ligamentum arteriosum that forms when the ductus closes.

Normal Anatomy

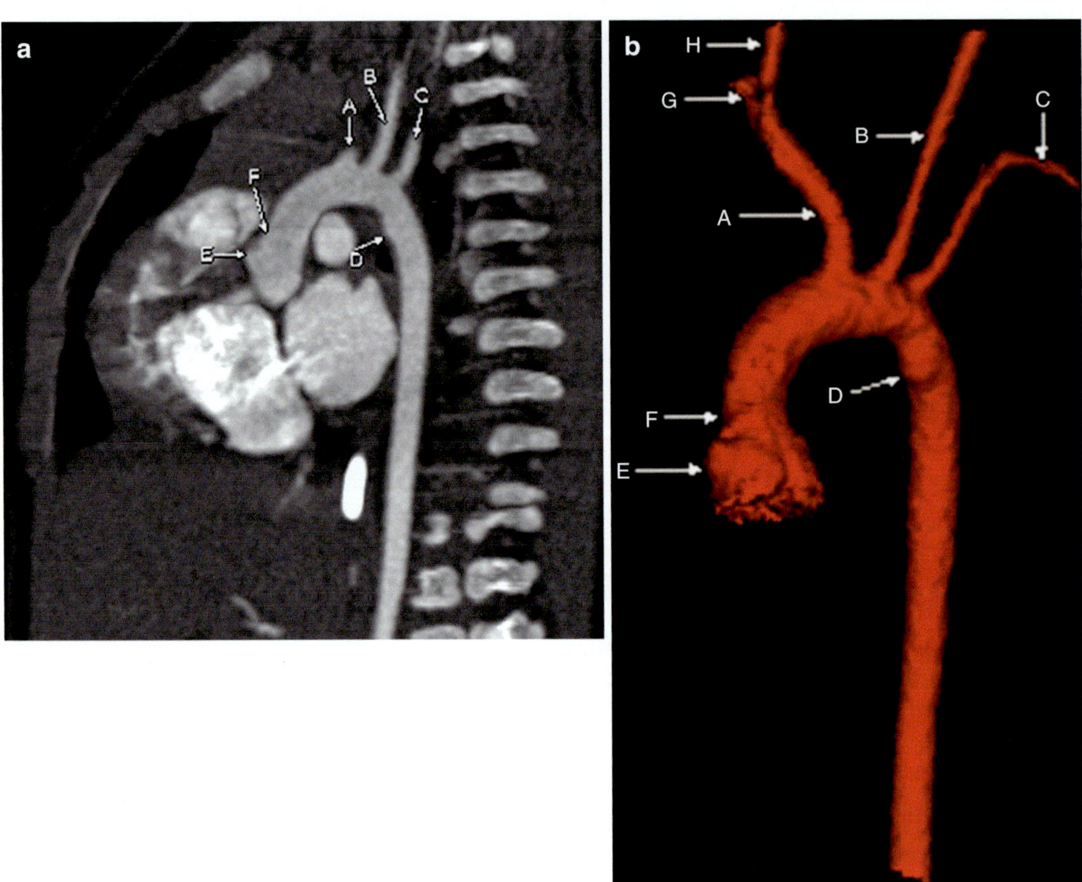

Fig. 7.1 Sagittal maximum-intensity projection (MIP; **a**) and lateral projection color-coded three-dimensional (3D; **b**) images from a cardiac CTA demonstrating a normal three-vessel aortic arch. The sinus of Valsalva (*E*) typically bulges, with immediate narrowing at the sinotubular junction (*F*). The first vessel of a left aortic arch is the right brachiocephalic artery (*A*), which divides further into right subclavian (*G*) and right common carotid (*H*) arteries. The second vessel off the arch is the left common carotid artery (*B*) and the last is the left subclavian artery (*C*). Notice the typical ductus bump (*D*), which is seen along the undersurface of the descending aortic arch

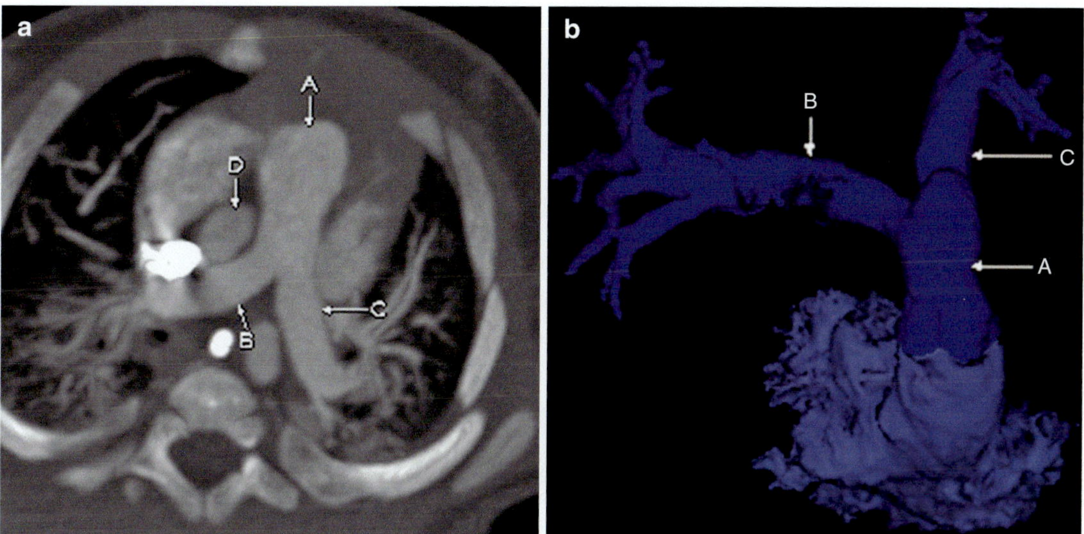

Fig. 7.2 Axial MIP (**a**) and 3D color-coded (**b**) images from a cardiac CTA. The main (*A*), right (*B*), and left (*C*) pulmonary arteries are shown. Notice the normal position of the ascending aorta (*D*) posterior to and to the right of the pulmonary outflow tract

PDA

PDA is the persistence of the normal prenatal vascular connection between the pulmonary artery and proximal descending aorta or brachiocephalic artery. In utero, the ductus arteriosus functions as a right-to-left shunt to bypass the pulmonary vasculature. After birth, it becomes a left-to-right shunt because of the higher pressures in the aorta relative to those in the pulmonary system. A PDA is a type of acyanotic heart disease with increased pulmonary vasculature, cardiomegaly, and a prominent "ductus bump." A longstanding PDA may cause pulmonary hypertension, flow reversal, and cyanosis (Eisenmenger's physiology). When it closes, a PDA forms a ligamentum arteriosum, which often calcifies.

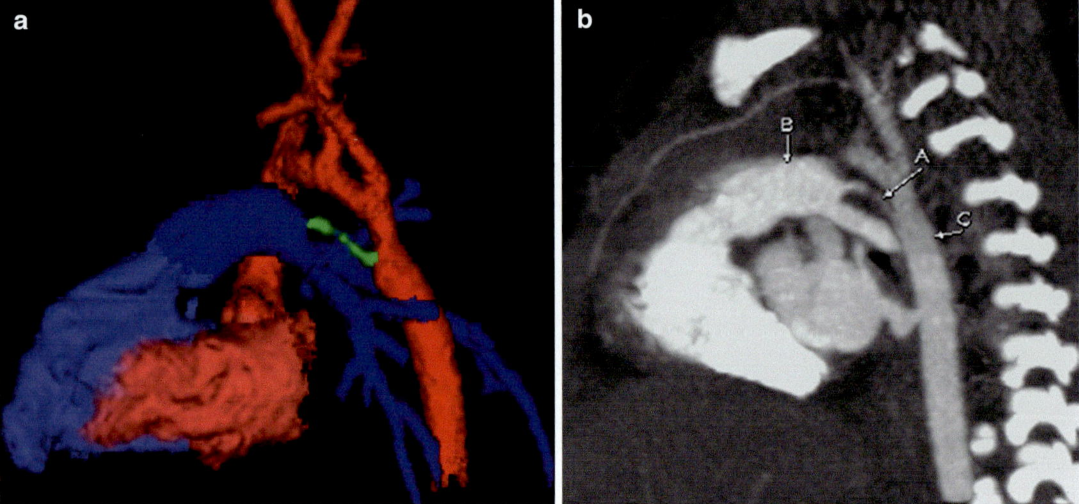

Fig. 7.3 Color-coded 3D (**a**) and sagittal MIP (**b**) images from a cardiac CT showing a small PDA (*green*, *A*) connecting the pulmonary artery (*blue*, *B*) to the proximal descending aorta (*red*, *C*)

PDA from the Left Brachiocephalic Artery

A PDA may arise from the aorta or left brachiocephalic/left subclavian artery. With a right arch and an aberrant subclavian artery, the PDA may complete a vascular ring when it arises from an aberrant left subclavian artery.

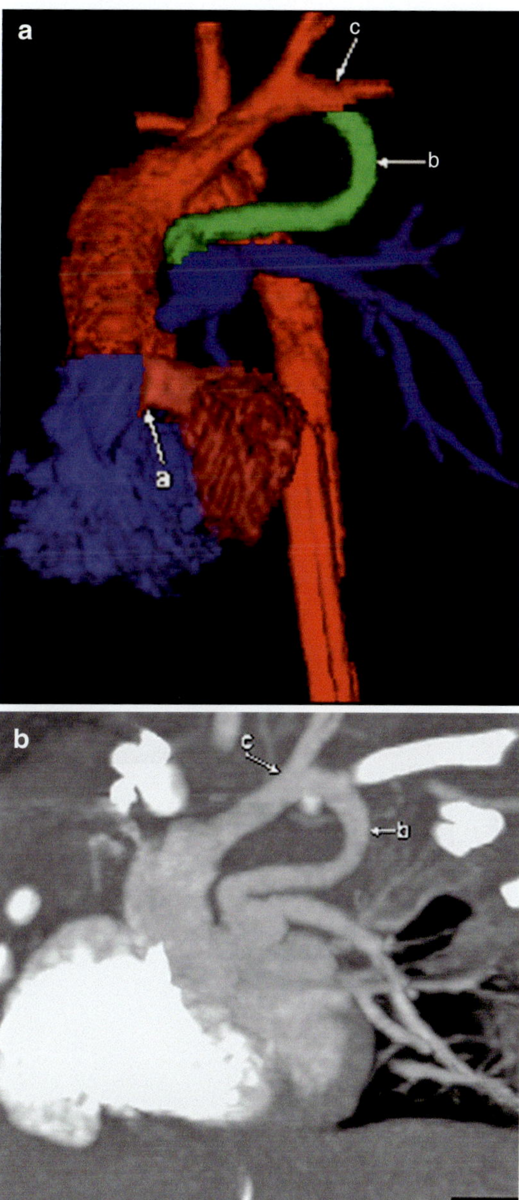

Fig. 7.4 Color-coded 3D (**a**) and sagittal MIP (**b**) images from a cardiac CT showing a PDA (*b*) attached to the left subclavian artery (*c*) in a patient with a right aortic arch. A ventricular septal defect (VSD; *a*) also is shown on the 3D image

PDA from the Descending Aortic Arch

A PDA often is necessary for survival, especially if there is obstruction to aortic flow, as seen in severe aortic stenosis, coarctation of the aorta, interruption of the aortic arch, and hypoplastic left ventricle. The PDA may be stented (hybrid procedure) in some patients with hypoplastic left ventricle.

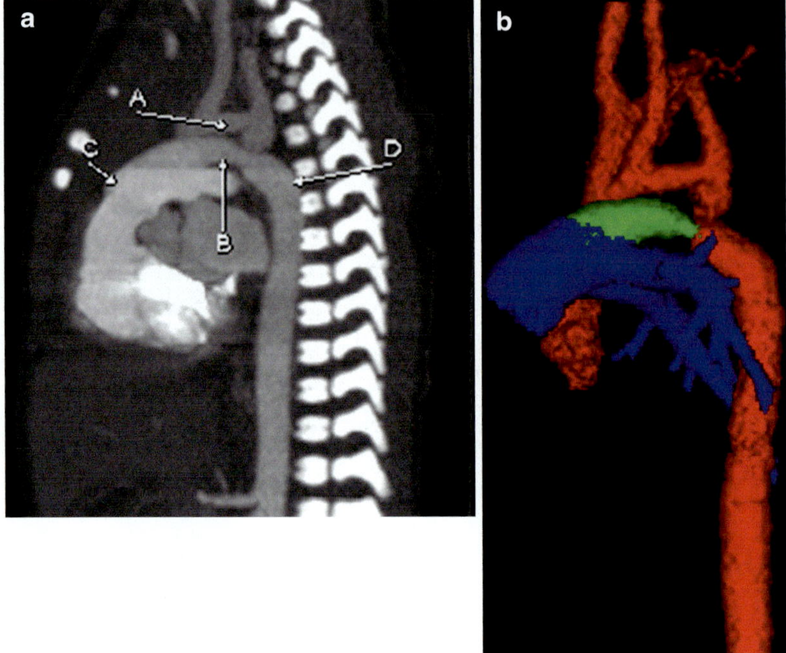

Fig. 7.5 Sagittal MIP (**a**) and color-coded 3D (**b**) images from a cardiac CT scan showing a PDA (*B*, *green*) connecting the descending aortic arch (*D*, *red*) and the pulmonary artery (*C*, *blue*). A hypoplastic aortic arch (*A*, *red*) also is shown

Bilateral PDA

Rarely, a PDA may be separate and bilateral, arising from the left brachiocephalic artery and aorta. In these cases, the patient typically has complex congenital heart disease with several other anomalies.

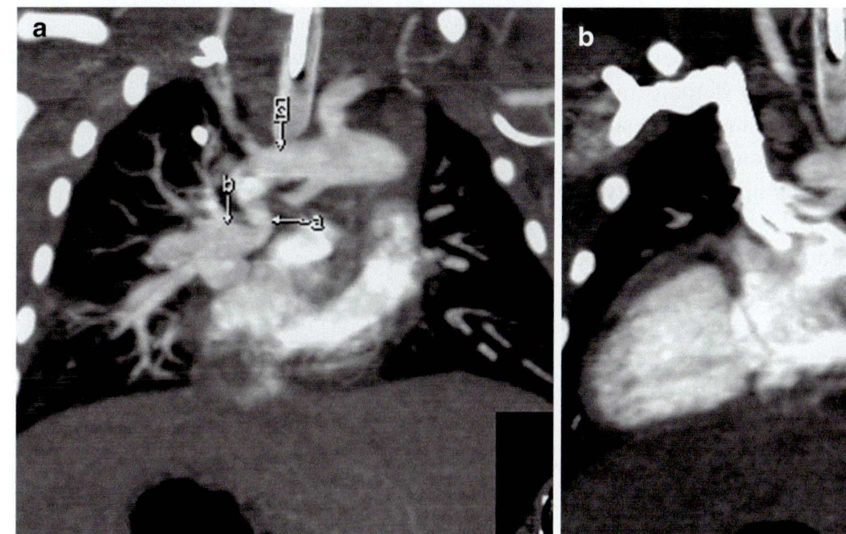

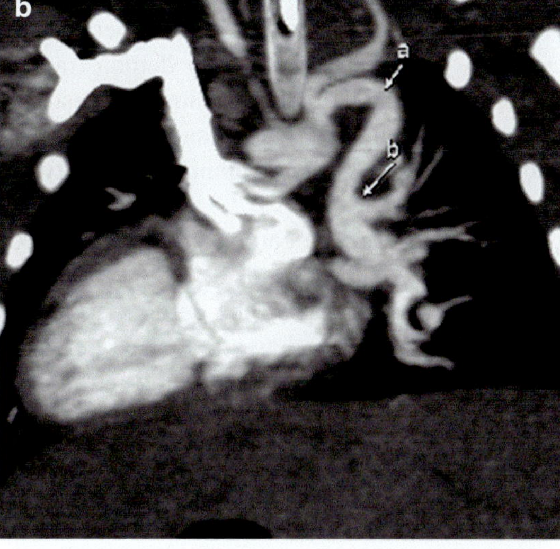

Fig. 7.6 (**a**) MIP image from a cardiac CT demonstrating a PDA (*a*) extending from the aortic arch (*c*) to give rise to the right pulmonary artery (*b*). (**b**) Coronal MIP image showing a second, tortuous PDA (*a*) from the descending aortic arch, giving rise to the left pulmonary artery (*b*)

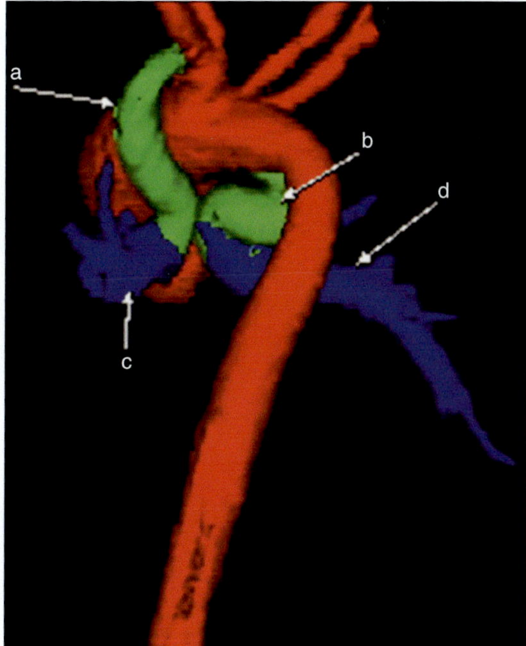

Fig. 7.7 Color-coded 3D image from a cardiac CT scan showing bilateral PDAs (*a* and *b*) giving rise to the right (*d*) and left (*c*) pulmonary arteries

Aortic Atresia

Aortic atresia is part of the hypoplastic left heart syndrome and involves hypoplasia/atresia of the ascending aorta, aortic valve, left ventricle, and mitral valve. Patients depend on a PDA for survival; death occurs within days (as the PDA closes) if the condition is untreated. Patients have cyanosis, with chest radiography demonstrating cardiomegaly and pulmonary venous congestion. Echocardiography, CT, MRI, and angiography may be used for treatment planning. A variety of surgical options exist.

In aortic atresia, the coronary arteries receive retrograde blood flow from the PDA up to the aortic arch and then down the coronary arteries via a hypoplastic ascending aorta. The brain and upper extremities also depend on the retrograde flow from the PDA.

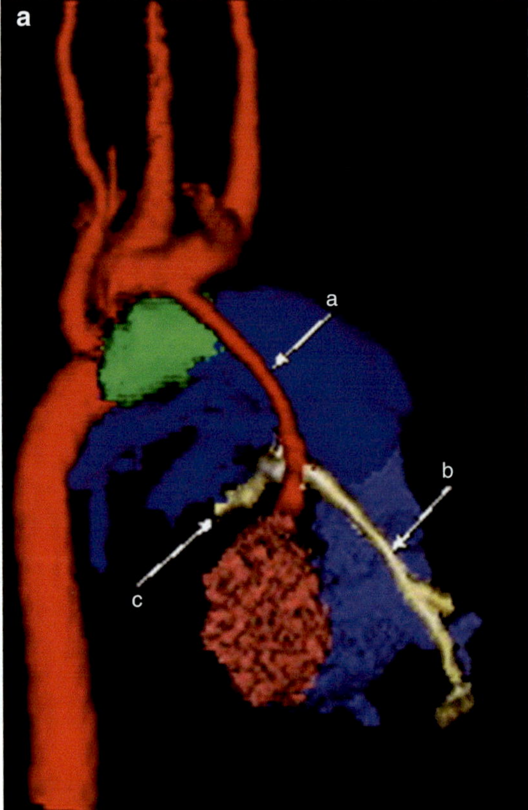

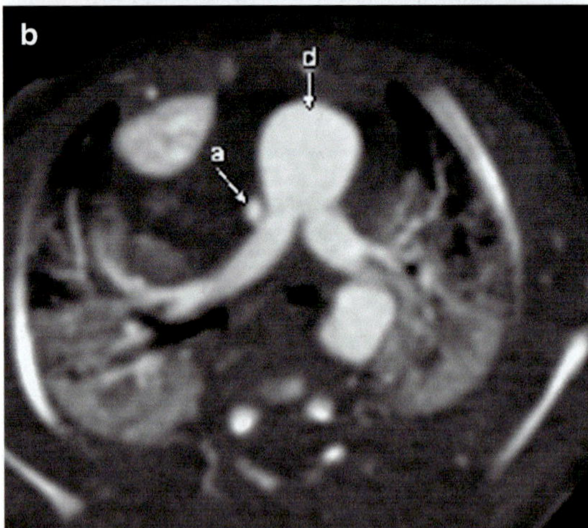

Fig. 7.8 3D color-coded (**a**) and axial (**b**) images demonstrating hypoplasia of the ascending aorta (*a*). The main pulmonary artery (*d*, *blue*) provides blood flow through a PDA (*green*), allowing retrograde flow to the great vessels coming off the arch (*red*) and the coronary arteries (*tan*, *b* and *c*)

Aortic Stenosis

Aortic stenosis may be valvular, subvalvular, or supravalvular (Williams syndrome). In neonates/infants, chest radiography is normal or shows mild cardiomegaly and pulmonary edema. In children/adolescents, chest radiography is often normal, even if the aortic stenosis is severe. Patients with aortic stenosis have thickening with fusion of the aortic valve leaflets, poststenotic dilatation of the ascending aorta, a systolic flow jet into the ascending aorta, and left ventricular hypertrophy. MRI and echocardiography may be used to assess the transvalvular pressure gradient, the regurgitant fraction, and ventricular function.

Valvular Aortic Stenosis

Valvular aortic stenosis, reported in 1–2 % of the population, most commonly is the result of a bicuspid aortic valve, although bicuspid aortic valves do not always cause significant stenosis. It is more common in males and has a familial predilection.

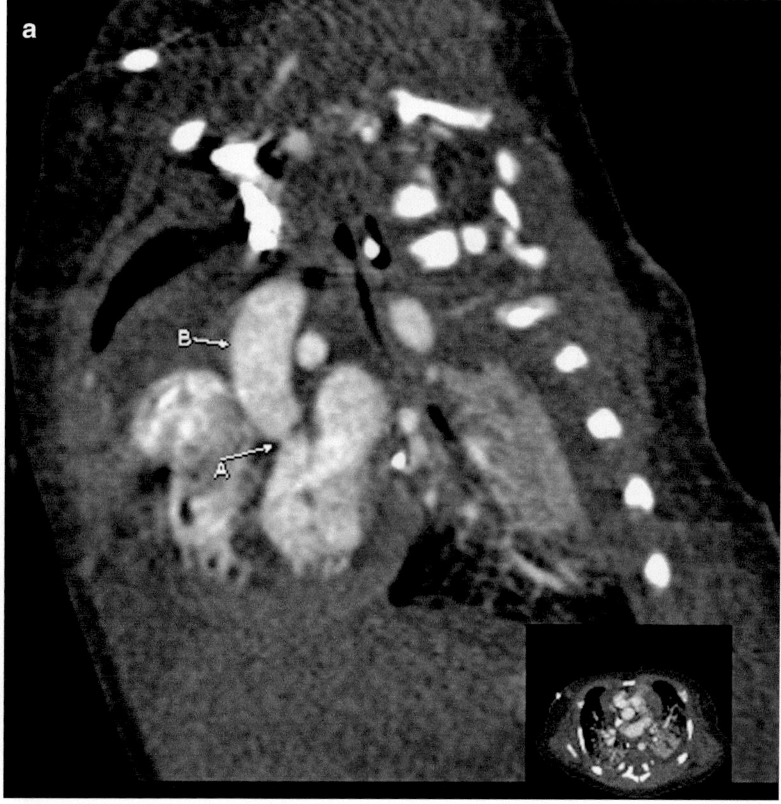

Fig. 7.9 Sagittal (**a**) and axial (**b**) contrast-enhanced cardiac CT images demonstrating narrowing of the aorta at the level of the aortic valve (*A*) with thickening of the bicuspid valve leaflets (*A*). Poststenotic dilatation of the ascending aorta (*B*) also is seen

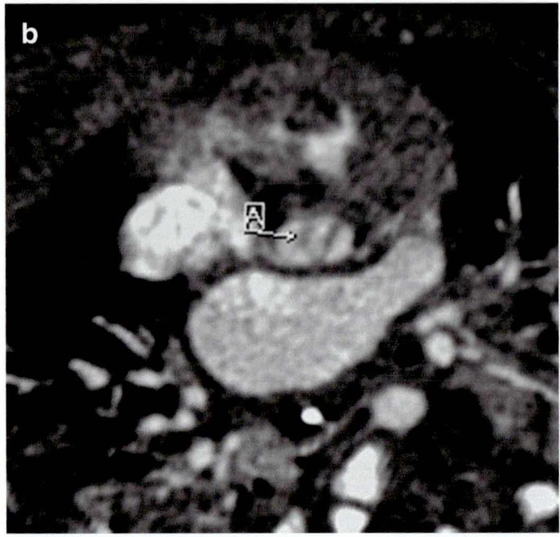

Fig. 7.9 (continued)

Supravalvular Aortic Stenosis (Williams Syndrome)

Supravalvular aortic stenosis occurs above the aortic valve, giving the proximal aorta an "hourglass" appearance. It is associated with stenosis of other vessels, such as the pulmonary and coronary arteries and descending abdominal aorta. Children with this disease may have elf-like facial features and mental retardation.

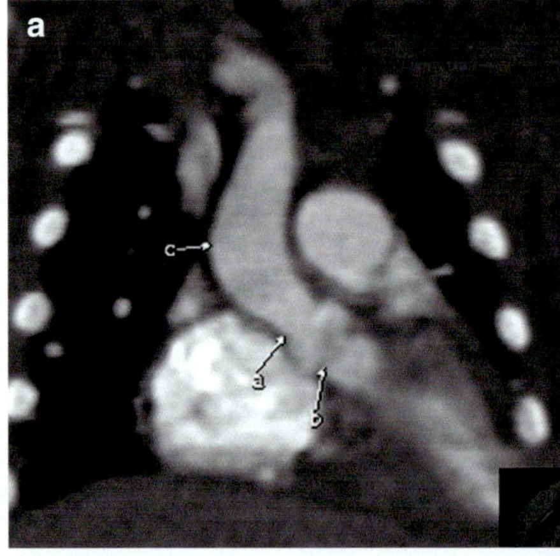

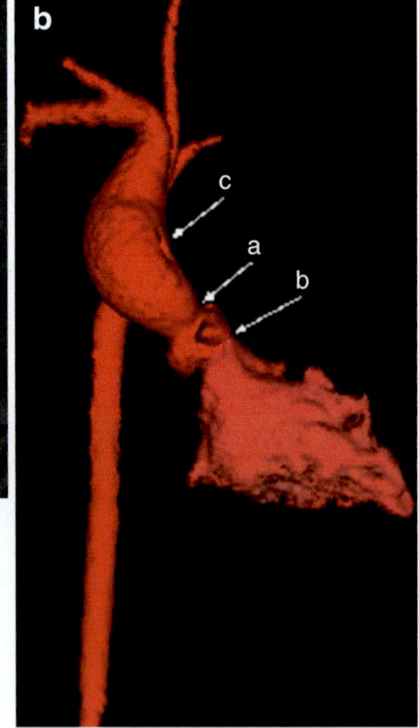

Fig. 7.10 Coronal MIP (**a**) and color-coded 3D (**b**) images from a cardiac CT scan in a patient with Williams syndrome. The images show supravalvar aortic stenosis (*a*) with poststenotic dilatation (*c*) of the aorta. Notice that the subvalvular region is of normal caliber (*b*). The contours of the ascending aorta often are described as hourglass shaped

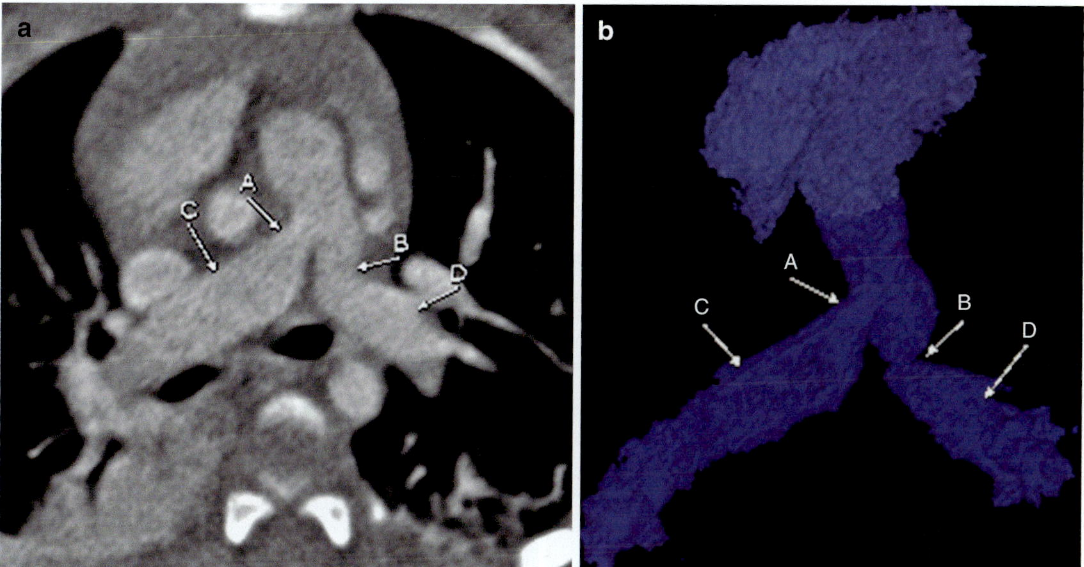

Fig. 7.11 Axial (**a**) and color-coded 3D (**b**) images in a patient with known Williams syndrome. The images demonstrate stenosis of the proximal left (*B*) and right (*A*) pulmonary arteries with associated poststenotic dilatation (*C* and *D*). Pulmonic stenosis is a common finding in patients with Williams syndrome

Hypertrophic Cardiomyopathy with Subaortic Stenosis

Hypertrophic cardiomyopathy with subaortic stenosis, the most common form of cardiomyopathy in children, is marked by thickening of the interventricular septum, causing left ventricular outflow tract obstruction (LVOT). The etiology may be idiopathic. Infants of diabetic mothers also may develop significant hypertrophy of the interventricular septum and may have subvalvular stenosis.

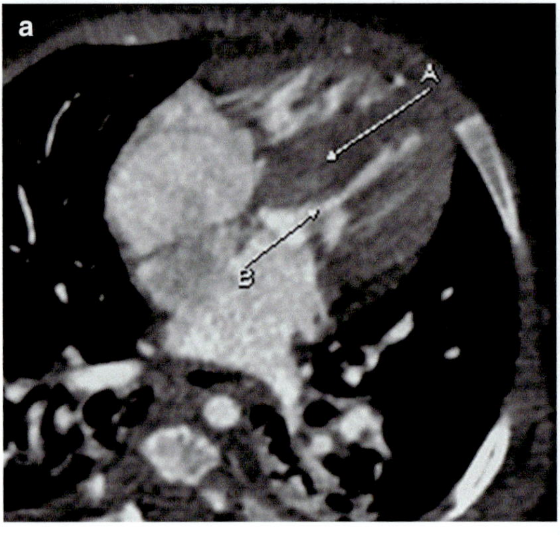

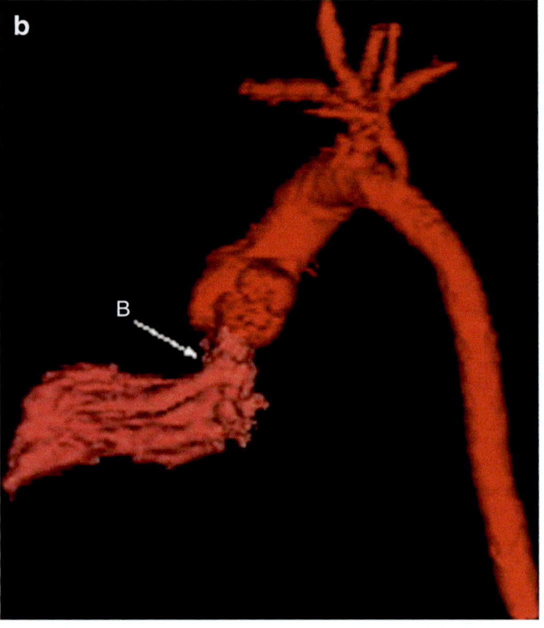

Fig. 7.12 Axial contrast-enhanced CT image through the heart (**a**) and corresponding color-coded 3D image (**b**) demonstrating severe thickening of the myocardial septum (*A*) and the free wall of the left ventricle, which results in narrowing of the aortic outflow tract (*B*) in the subvalvular region

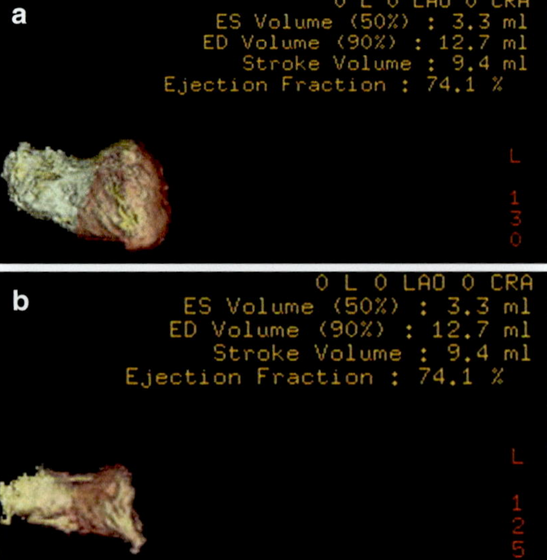

Fig. 7.13 Functional end-diastolic (**a**) and end-systolic (**b**) images from a cardiac CTA scan showing hyperdynamic function of the left ventricle with an ejection fraction of 74.1 % in a patient with hypertrophic cardiomyopathy

Pulmonic Stenosis

Pulmonic stenosis may be valvular (>90 % of cases) or supravalvular, or occur at the branches of the distal pulmonary arteries. Patients with this disease have a thickened, stenotic valve with poststenotic dilatation of the pulmonary artery. There is associated right ventricular hypertrophy. Heart size is normal, with a dilated main pulmonary artery segment. The clinical presentation is determined by the severity of stenosis and ranges from asymptomatic to severely cyanotic in infancy. Pulmonic stenosis is associated with Noonan syndrome, Williams syndrome, tetralogy of Fallot (TOF), Ellaville syndrome, and congenital rubella.

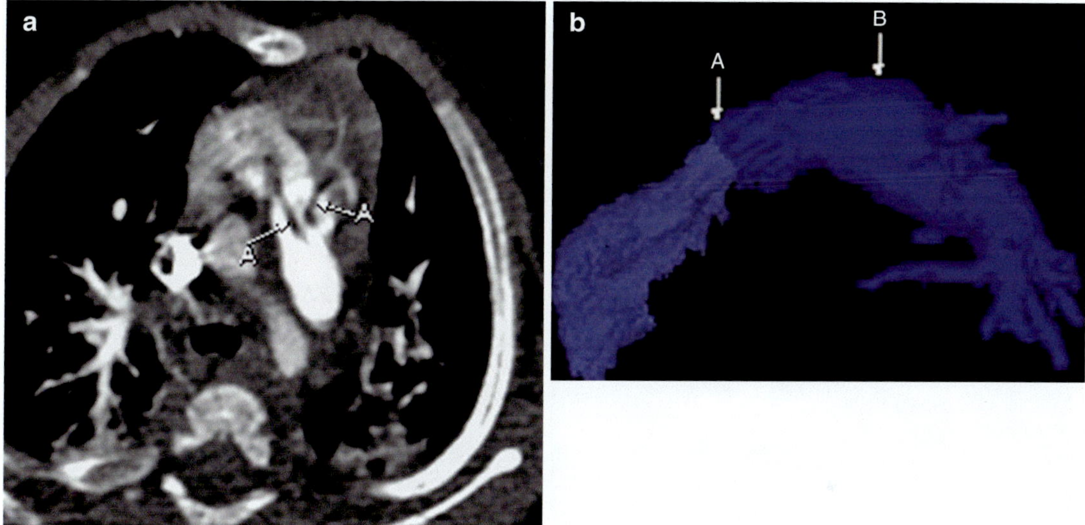

Fig. 7.14 Axial MIP (**a**) and color-coded (**b**) images from a cardiac CT scan demonstrating thickening and stenosis of the pulmonic valve (*A*) with associated poststenotic dilatation of the main pulmonary artery (*B*)

Dextro-Type Transposition of the Great Vessels

In dextro-transposition of the great vessels (DTGA), the aorta arises from the right ventricle and the pulmonary artery from the left ventricle. There is ventriculoarterial discordance with atrioventricular concordance. A shunt (PDA, VSD, atrial septal defect [ASD]) to mix oxygenated and deoxygenated blood is necessary for survival. The aortic valve is anterior to and to the left of the pulmonic valve. Chest radiography demonstrates a narrow mediastinum, cardiomegaly ("egg on a string"), and increased pulmonary vascularity. The right coronary artery typically arises from the noncoronary sinus in patients with DTGA. The coronary arteries typically arise from "facing" sinuses, meaning they arise from the coronary sinuses (noncoronary and left) facing the pulmonary artery.

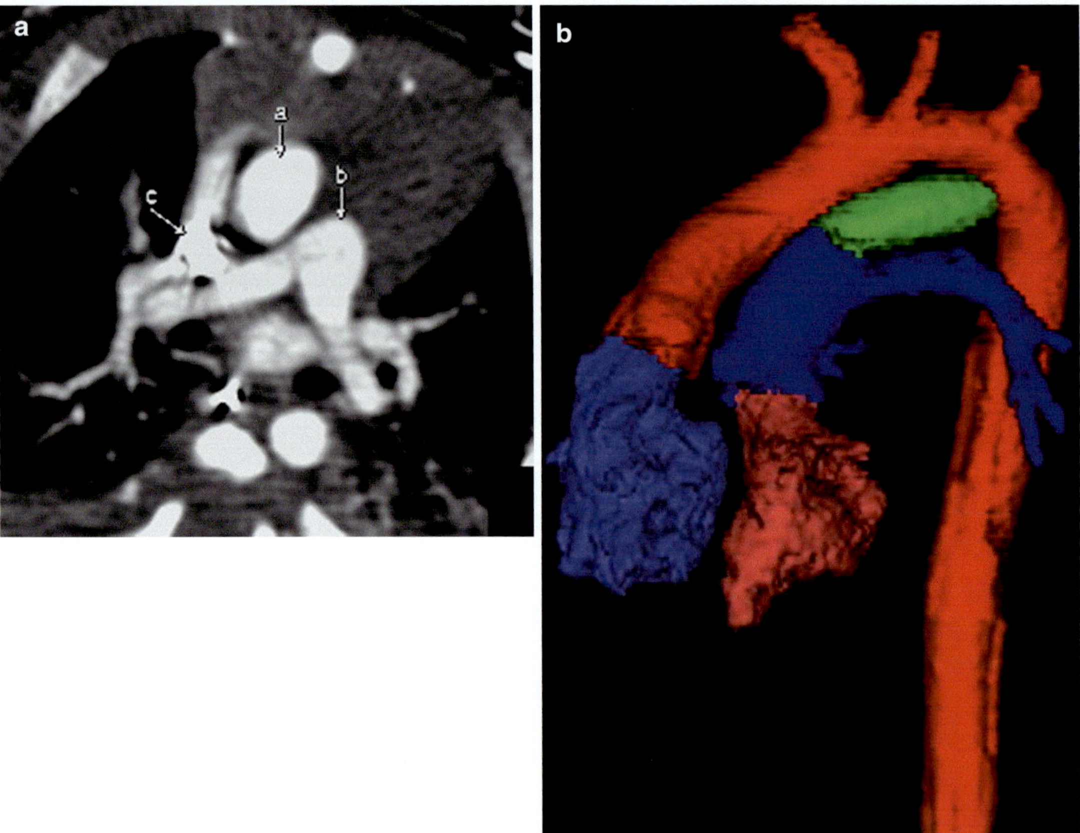

Fig. 7.15 (**a**) Axial MIP image from cardiac CT demonstrating the aortic root (*a*) anterior to and to the right of the pulmonary outflow tract (*b*). The SVC (*c*) is in the normal position. (**b**) Lateral view of a color-coded 3D image from a cardiac CT scan demonstrating the aorta (*red*) arising from the right ventricle (*purple*) while the pulmonary artery (*blue*) arises from the left ventricle (*salmon*) in this patient with DTGA. A PDA (*green*) is seen connecting the pulmonary artery (*blue*) to the aorta (*red*)

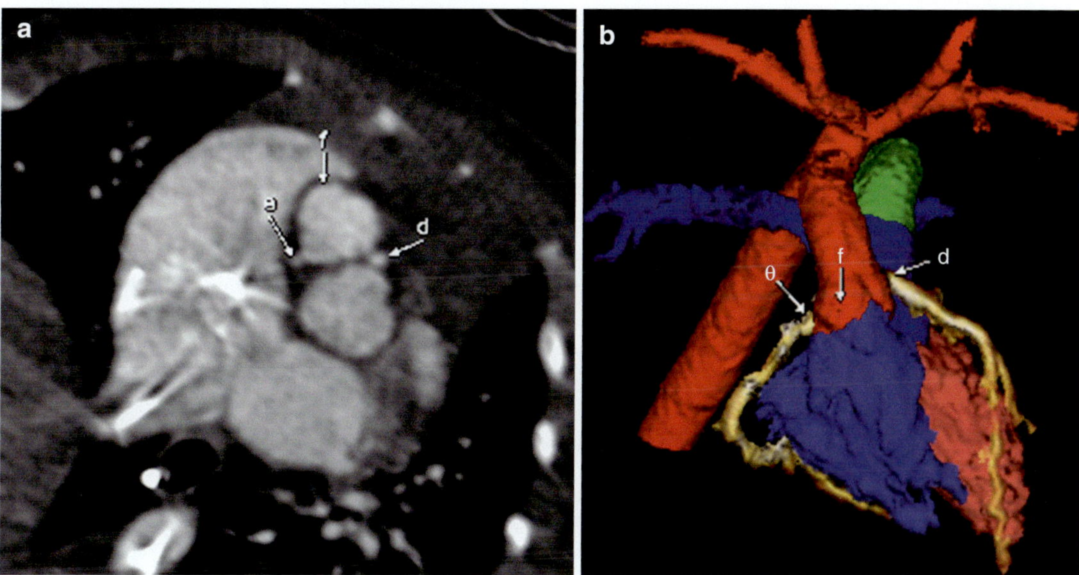

Fig. 7.16 Axial MIP (**a**) and color-coded 3D (**b**) images from a cardiac CT scan in a patient with DTGA showing the right coronary artery (*e*) arising from the noncoronary sinus and the left coronary artery (*d*) arising from the left coronary sinus. Notice that the right coronary sinus (*f*) is free of any coronary artery origin

Levo-Transposition of the Great Vessels

In levo-transposition, the great vessels and ventricles are inverted and there is atrioventricular and ventriculoarterial discordance. Right-sided blood flow is as follows: inferior/superior vena cava → right atrium → mitral valve → morphologic left ventricle (on right) → pulmonary circulation. Left-sided flow is as follows: pulmonary veins → left atrium → tricuspid valve → morphologic right ventricle (on left) → systemic circulation. The term *congenitally corrected transposition* is applied if there are no associated abnormalities (1 % of cases). The most common associated abnormalities include VSD (60–70 %) and LVOT obstruction (30–50 %). Chest radiography often demonstrates a straight left heart border.

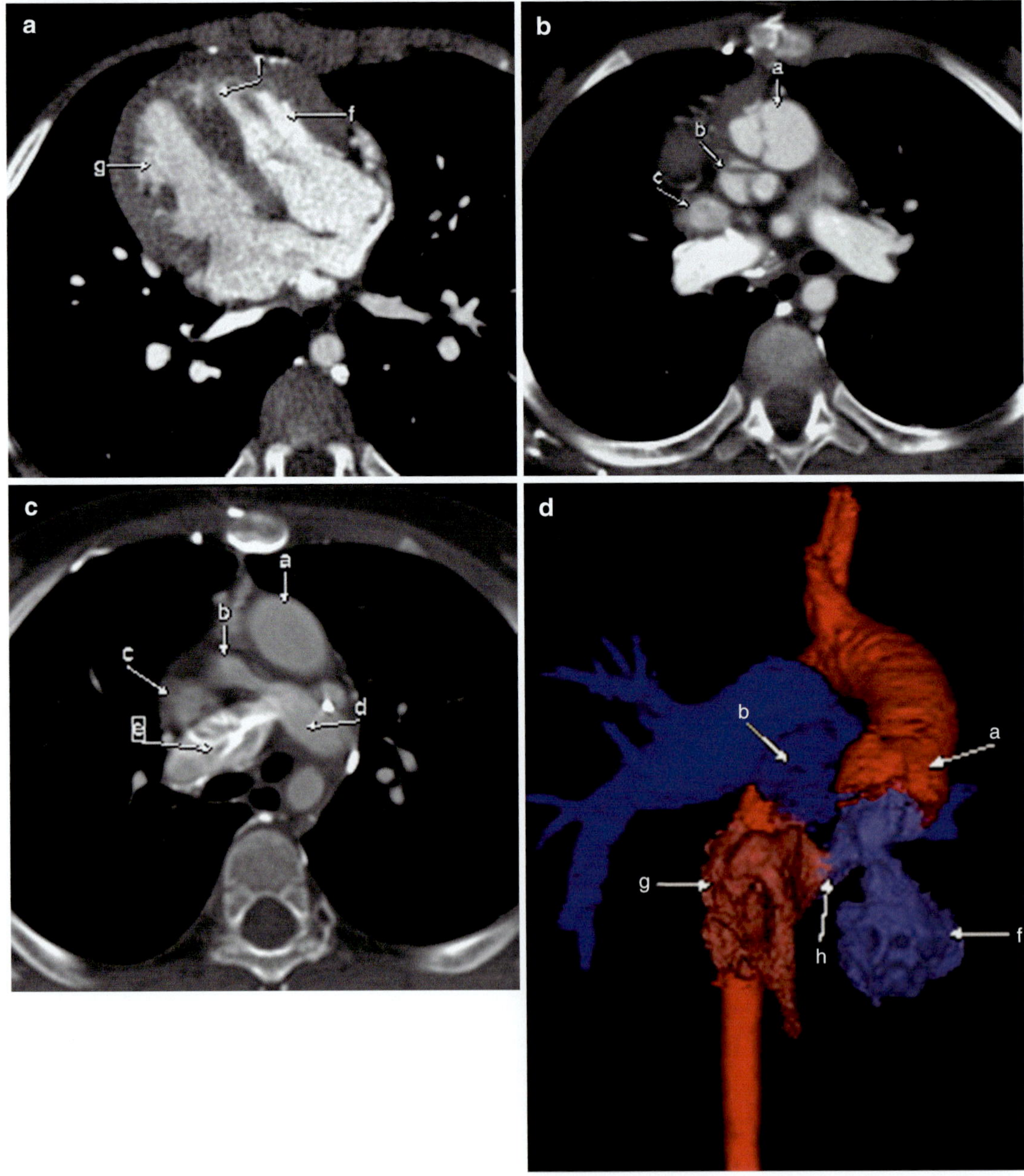

Double-Outlet Right Ventricle

In double-outlet right ventricle, the aorta and pulmonary artery arise completely or predominantly from the morphologic right ventricle. It often is part of complex heart disease. There are 16 variations based on the positioning of the great arteries and VSD; the most common is subaortic VSD with normal positioning of the great vessels. The radiographic appearance depends on the physiology of the lesion. Patients with double-outlet right ventricle have mild cardiomegaly and decreased pulmonary vasculature, often similar in appearance to TOF.

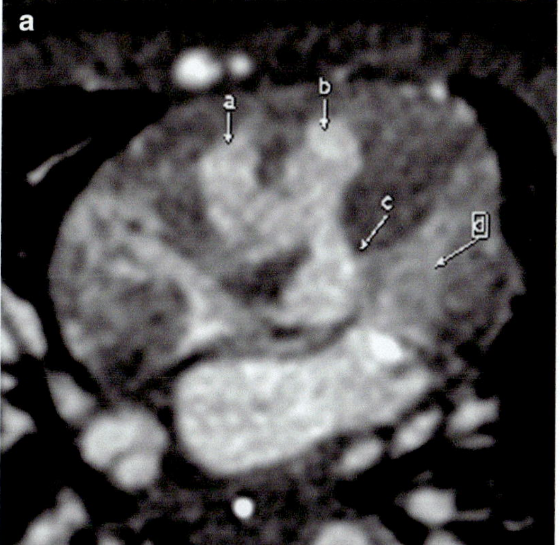

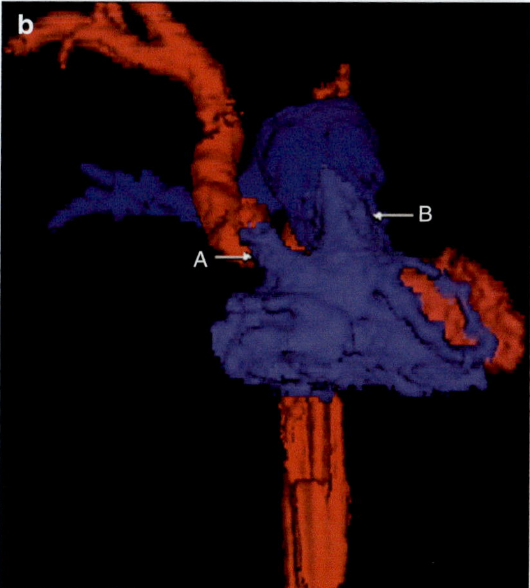

Fig. 7.18 Axial MIP image from cardiac CT (**a**) and anterior view of a color-coded 3D reconstruction (**b**) demonstrating the aorta outflow (*a*, *A*) to the right of the main pulmonary outflow (*b*, *B*), with both arising from the right ventricle (*purple*). A VSD (*c*) also is seen connecting the right and left (*d*) ventricles

Fig. 7.17 Three contrast-enhanced axial cardiac CT images (**a–c**) and corresponding color-coded 3D image (**d**) showing the morphologic left ventricle (*g*) positioned on the right with a relatively smooth wall. The morphologic right ventricle (*f*) is on the left and can be identified by its trabeculated wall and moderator band (*l*). The aorta (*a*) arises from the morphologic right ventricle and lies anterior to and to the left of the pulmonary artery (*b*), which arises from the morphologic left ventricle. The right (*e*) and left (*d*) pulmonary arteries, along with the superior vena cava (*c*), are seen on the axial images. The 3D image demonstrates a VSD (*h*), which is present in 60–70 % of levo-transposition cases

Hypoplastic-Type Coarctation of the Aorta

Hypoplastic coarctation of the aorta also has been referred to as *preductal* or *infantile-type coarctation*. In infants with this condition, no significant collaterals have had time to develop. Patients with severe coarctation often present in infancy with heart failure once the PDA closes. Heart size is normal in these patients as long as the ventricular hypertrophy can overcome the stenosis.

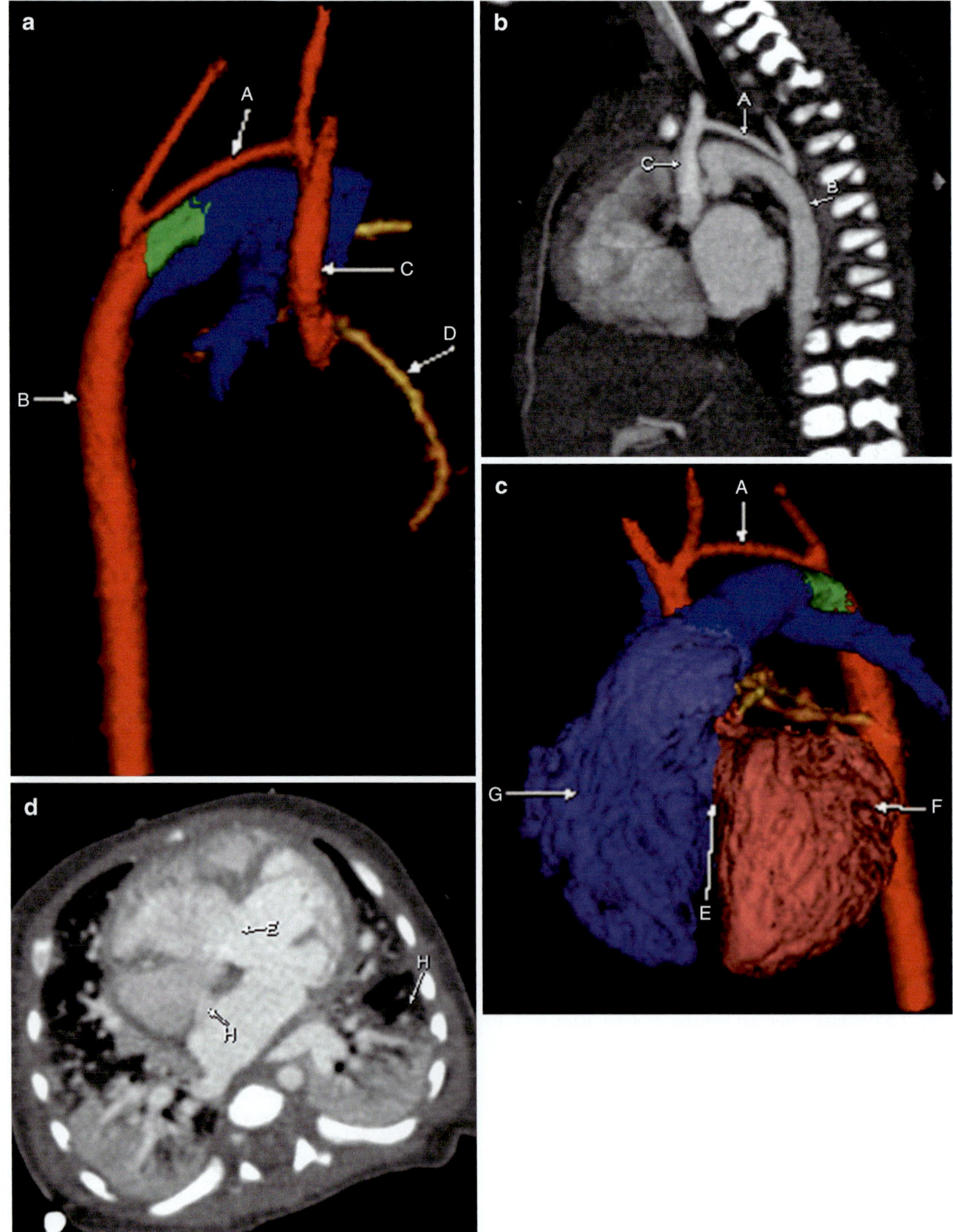

Focal-Type Coarctation of the Aorta

In focal coarctation, there is focal obstruction of the descending aortic arch, which may be preductal, juxtaductal, or postductal. This condition typically presents in older children and adolescents. Collateral vessels are common. Chest radiography demonstrates a normal heart size and pulmonary vasculature with dilatation of the descending aorta from poststenotic dilatation. On plain x-ray film, this forms a figure "3" sign. Rib notching is seen from the large collateral vessels.

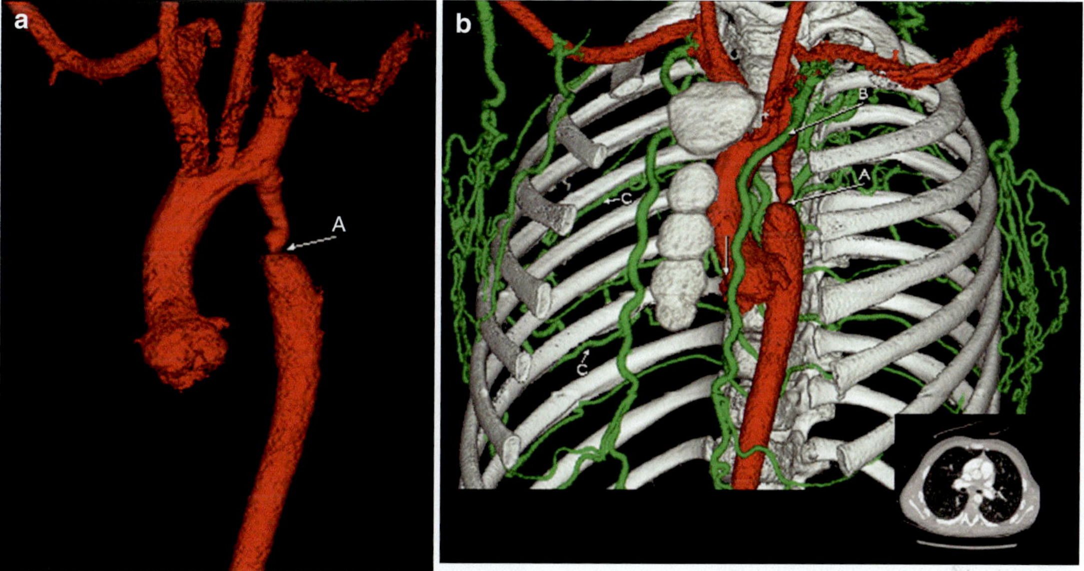

Fig. 7.20 Color-coded 3D (**a** and **b**) and sagittal (**c**) MIP images from cardiac CT showing a focal stenosis (*A*) of the descending aortic arch with multiple enlarged collateral vessels, including internal mammary (*B*) and intercostal arteries (*C*)

Fig. 7.19 Lateral (**a**) and oblique (**c**) projection color-coded 3D models and sagittal (**b**) and axial (**d**) MIP images from a cardiac CTA scan demonstrating a severely hypoplastic-type coarctation (*A*) of the transverse aortic arch proximal to the origin of the left subclavian artery. Notice that the descending aorta (*B*) is fed by a PDA (*green*). There is some hypoplasia of the ascending aorta (*C*), with the right coronary artery (*D*) arising from the right coronary sinus. A large VSD (*E*) is noted between the right (*G*) and left (*F*) ventricles, with a secundum-type ASD (*H*, heart) also seen. There is massive cardiomegaly and bilateral pulmonary edema (*H*, lungs), as this patient is in heart failure

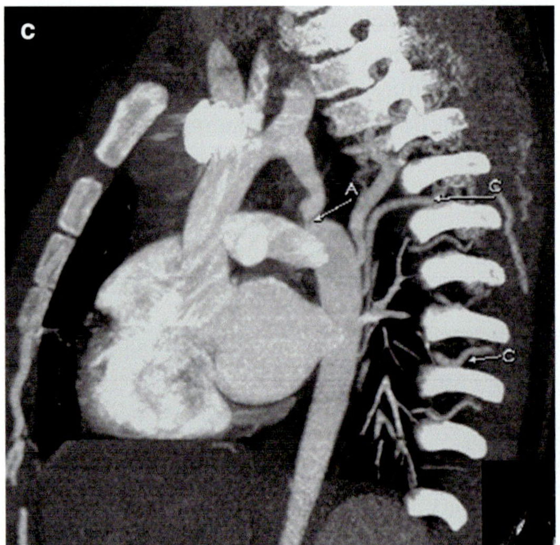

Fig. 7.20 (continued)

Pulmonic Atresia

Pulmonic atresia is marked by an imperforate pulmonary valve due to abnormal formation. A PDA or collaterals are necessary to provide blood flow to the pulmonary vessels. Patients with this condition have right ventricular hypoplasia with associated coronary artery abnormalities.

Pulmonic atresia may occur with or without a VSD; with a VSD, it is considered the most severe form of TOF. Imaging shows cardiomegaly and normal pulmonary vasculature.

Pulmonic Atresia with an Intact Ventricular Septum and Right Ventricular Hypoplasia

In patients with pulmonic atresia with an intact ventricular septum and right ventricular hypoplasia, the right ventricle may be severely hypoplastic. Coronary artery fistulas (sinusoids) frequently are present. A PDA must be present with an ASD or a patent foramen ovale.

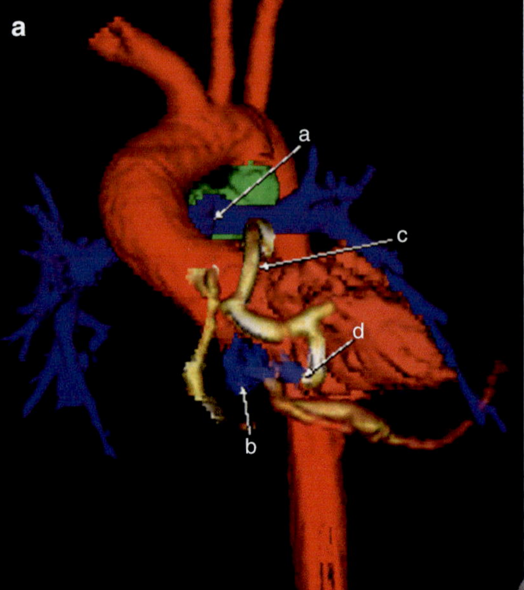

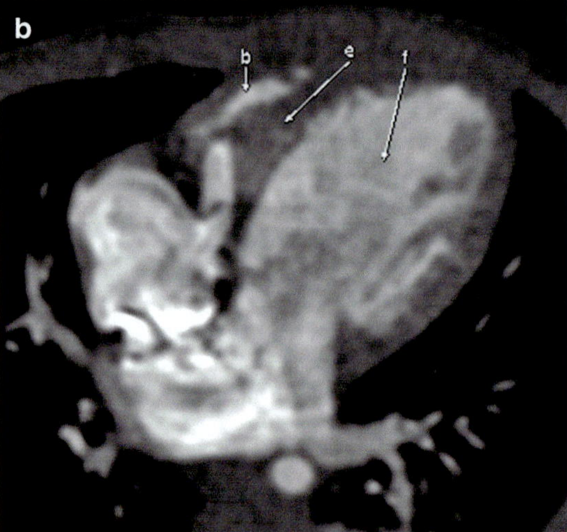

Fig. 7.21 Frontal color-coded 3D (**a**) and axial (**b**) images from a cardiac CT scan demonstrating right and left pulmonary arteries (*blue*) without direct attachment to the hypoplastic right ventricle (*b*) because of the long atretic segment (*a*) of the pulmonary artery. The left coronary artery is enlarged (*c*) and forms a fistula with the right ventricle (*d*). Notice that the interventricular septum is intact (*e*) and the left ventricle is enlarged (*f*)

Pulmonic Atresia with VSD, Type 1

In type 1 pulmonic atresia with VSD, most of the flow goes through the PDA to the pulmonary arteries. Some small collaterals may be present. Closure of the PDA is life threatening.

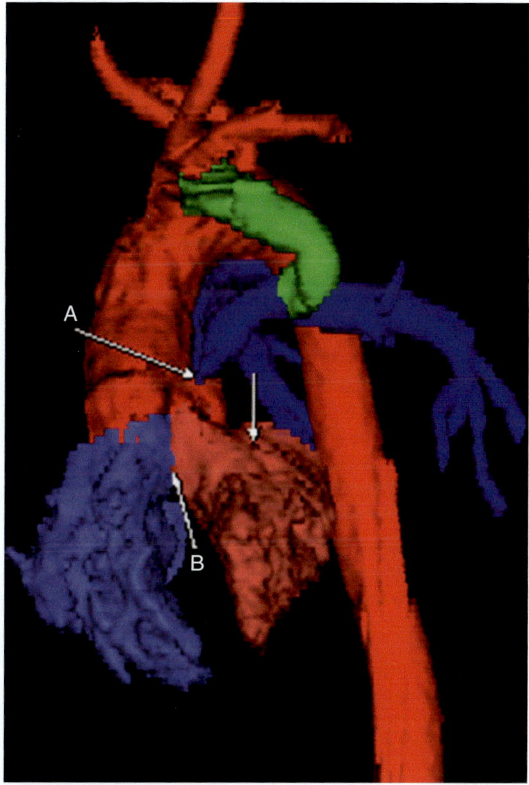

Fig. 7.22 3D color-coded image from a cardiac CT scan showing a VSD (*B*) connecting the left (*arrow*) and right (*purple*) ventricles with severe pulmonary artery stenosis (*A*). The pulmonary arteries receive blood flow from the PDA (*green*), and no other significant collateral flow is present

Pulmonic Atresia with VSD, Type 2

In type 2 pulmonic atresia with VSD, the flow from the pulmonary arteries and aortopulmonary collaterals is approximately equal. A PDA may be present. The pulmonary arteries are smaller than normal.

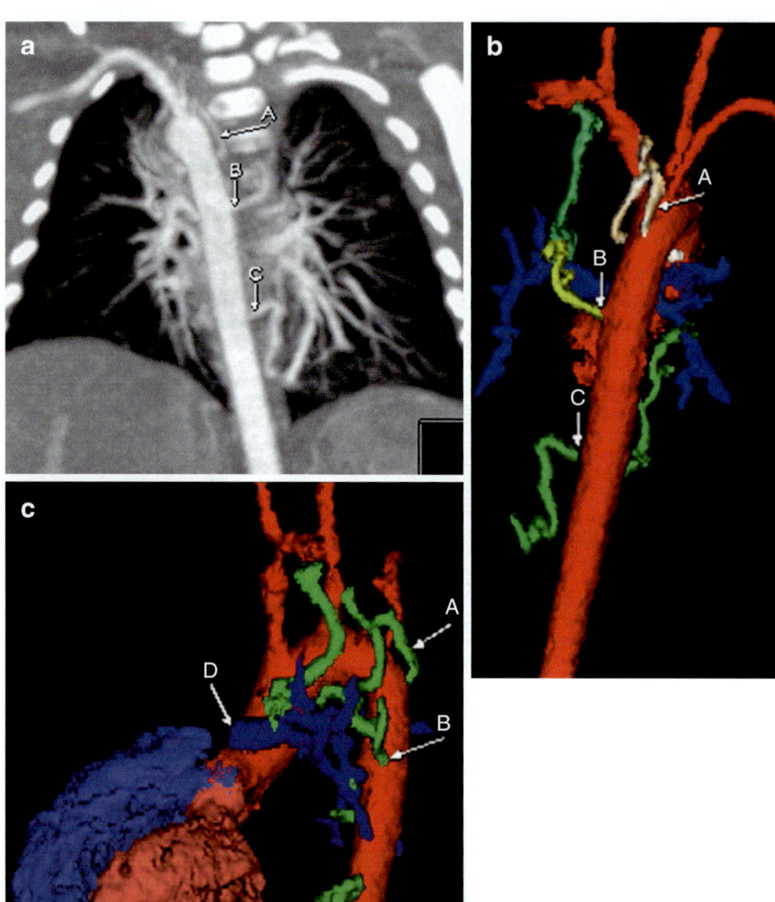

Fig. 7.23 Coronal MIP image (**a**) along with anterior (**b**) and lateral (**c**) color-coded 3D images from cardiac CT demonstrating multiple systemic-to-pulmonary collaterals (*A*, *B*, and *C*), which can provide blood flow to the pulmonary vasculature. The atretic segment is missing (*D*) between the main pulmonary artery and the right ventricle. Both native pulmonary arteries are only mildly hypoplastic

Pulmonic Atresia with VSD, Type 3

In type 3 pulmonic atresia with VSD, most of the pulmonary blood flow comes from the aortopulmonary collaterals. The pulmonary arteries are markedly hypoplastic and often difficult to identify.

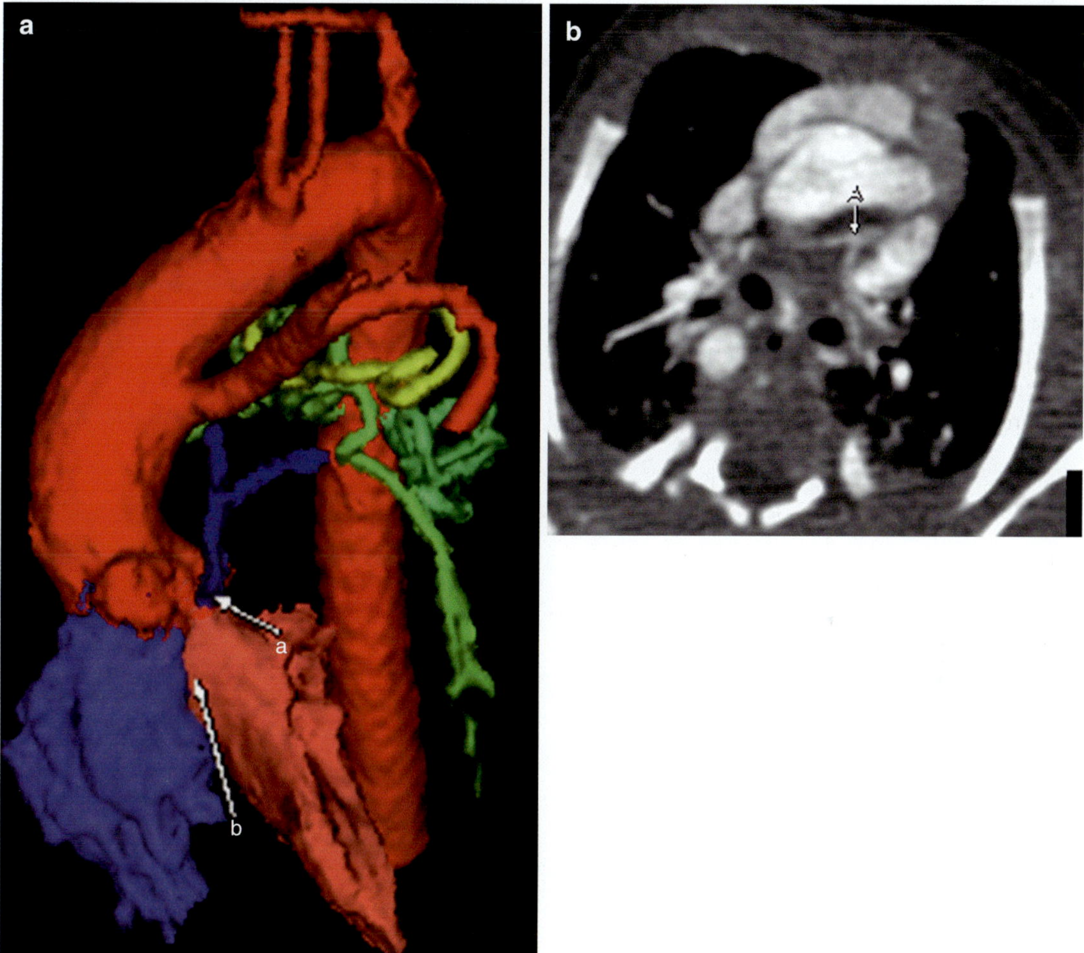

Fig. 7.24 Color-coded 3D (**a**) and axial contrast-enhanced (**b**) images from cardiac CT demonstrating markedly hypoplastic pulmonary arteries (*A*; *a*, *blue*) with an atretic proximal segment. Multiple collaterals (*green*, *yellow*) are necessary to provide blood flow to the lungs. A VSD (*b*) is shown

Interruption of the Aortic Arch

Interruption of the aortic arch is the absence or discontinuation of a portion of the aortic arch. Different types exist based on the location of the interruption: distal to the left subclavian artery origin (type A), between the left common carotid and left subclavian arteries (type B), or between the innominate and left common carotid arteries (type C). A PDA is necessary to oxygenate the lower extremities and abdominal organs. This condition often is associated with a VSD.

Interruption of the Aortic Arch, Type A

Type A interruption of the aortic arch occurs between the left subclavian artery and the descending aorta. Severe coarctation may be misinterpreted as this type of interruption.

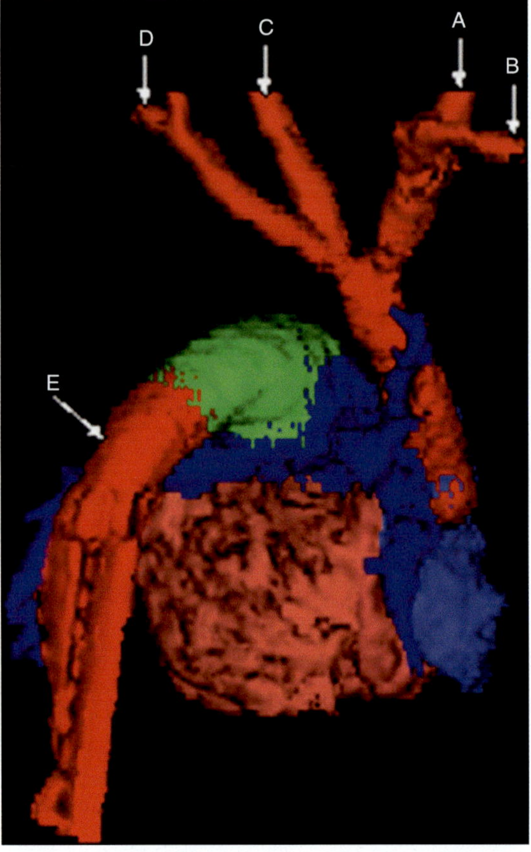

Fig. 7.25 Color-coded 3D image from cardiac CT demonstrating an interruption of the aortic arch distal to the left subclavian artery (*D*). The descending thoracic aorta is fed from a large PDA (*green*). The right common carotid (*A*), right subclavian (*B*), and left common carotid (*C*) arteries also are seen. Notice that the descending aorta (*E*) is supplied by the PDA (*green*)

Interruption of the Aortic Arch, Type B

Type B interruption is defined as an interruption of the aortic arch distal to the left common carotid artery and proximal to the left subclavian artery. It is the most common type of aortic arch interruption.

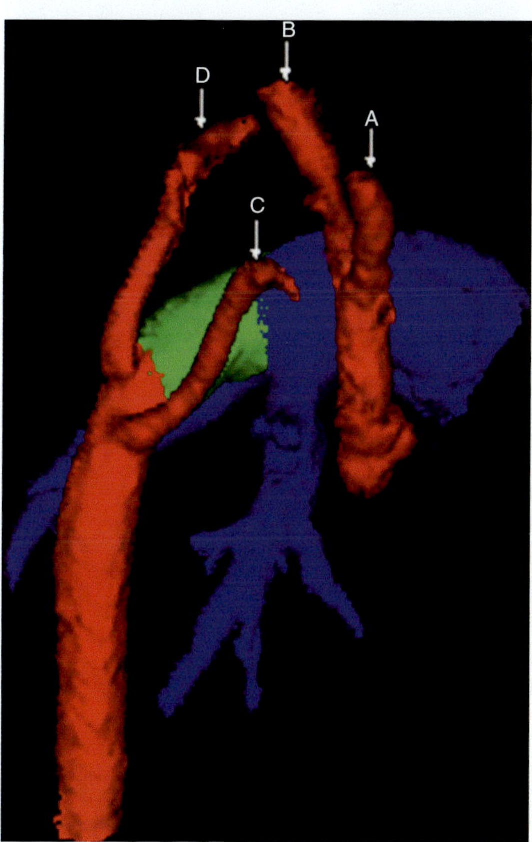

Fig. 7.26 Color-coded 3D image from a cardiac CT scan showing interruption of the aortic arch (*type B*) between the left common carotid (*B*) and left subclavian (*D*) arteries. Other vessels include the right common carotid (*A*) and aberrant right subclavian (*C*) arteries. Notice that the descending aorta and bilateral subclavian arteries (*D* and *C*) are supplied by the PDA (*green*)

Interruption of the Aortic Arch, Type C

Type C interruption is defined as an interruption of the aortic arch between the brachiocephalic and left common carotid arteries. It is the least common type of aortic arch interruption.

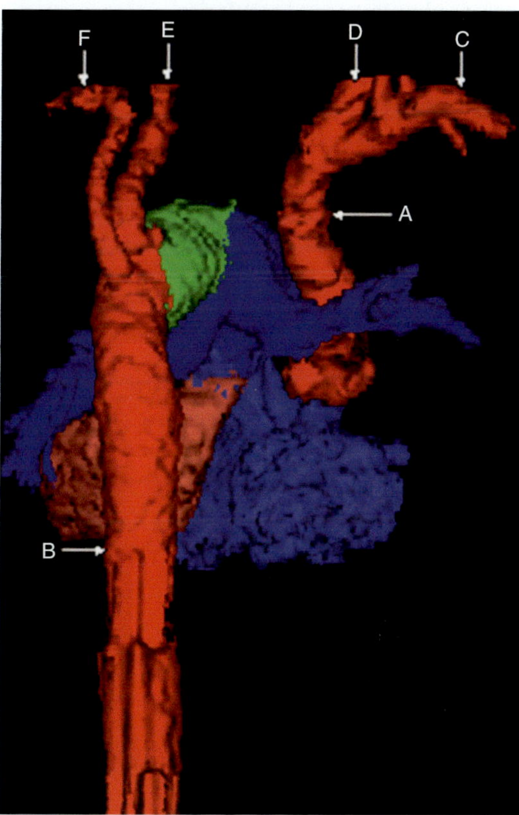

Fig. 7.27 3D color-coded image from cardiac CT demonstrating an interruption of the aortic arch (*type C*) between the innominate (*A*) and left common carotid (*E*) arteries. The left subclavian (*F*), right subclavian (*C*), and right common carotid (*D*) arteries also are displayed. Note that the PDA (*green*) gives rise to the descending thoracic aorta (*B*)

Truncus Arteriosus

In truncus arteriosus, a common arterial vessel arises from the heart and gives rise to the aorta, pulmonary artery, and coronary arteries. It is associated with right aortic arch in 30–40 % of cases. A high VSD exists immediately below the truncal valve. Imaging reveals cardiomegaly, increased pulmonary vascularity, a narrow mediastinum, and a right aortic arch. If untreated, truncus arteriosus leads to intractable heart failure. Classification schemes include the Van Praagh and the Collette and Edwards classifications.

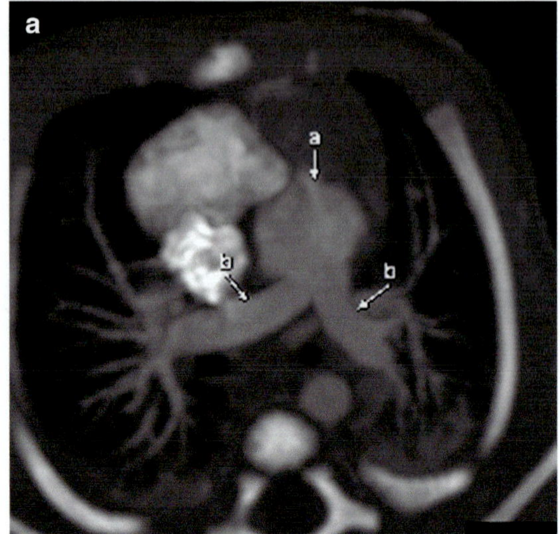

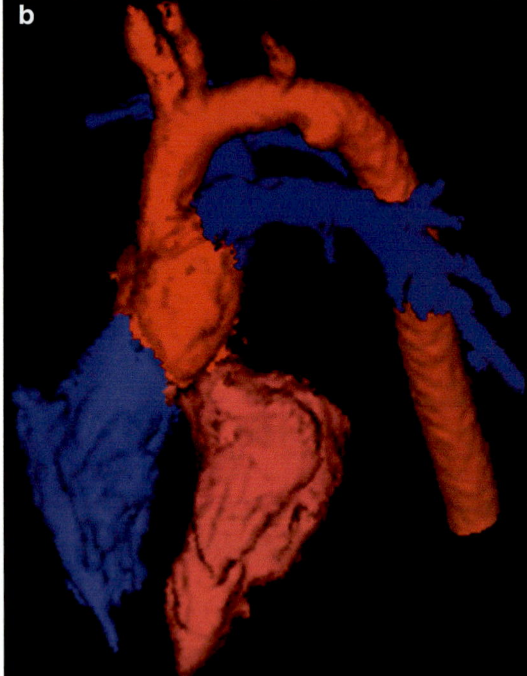

Fig. 7.28 Axial MIP (**a**) and lateral color-coded 3D (**b**) images from cardiac CT demonstrating a common truncus (*a*) giving rise to the right and left pulmonary arteries (*b*, *blue*) and the aorta (*red*)

Hemitruncus

In hemitruncus, one pulmonary artery arises from the aorta and the other is a continuation of the main pulmonary artery. Patients develop heart failure from the large left-to-right shunt. Chest radiography reveals increased pulmonary vascularity and cardiomegaly.

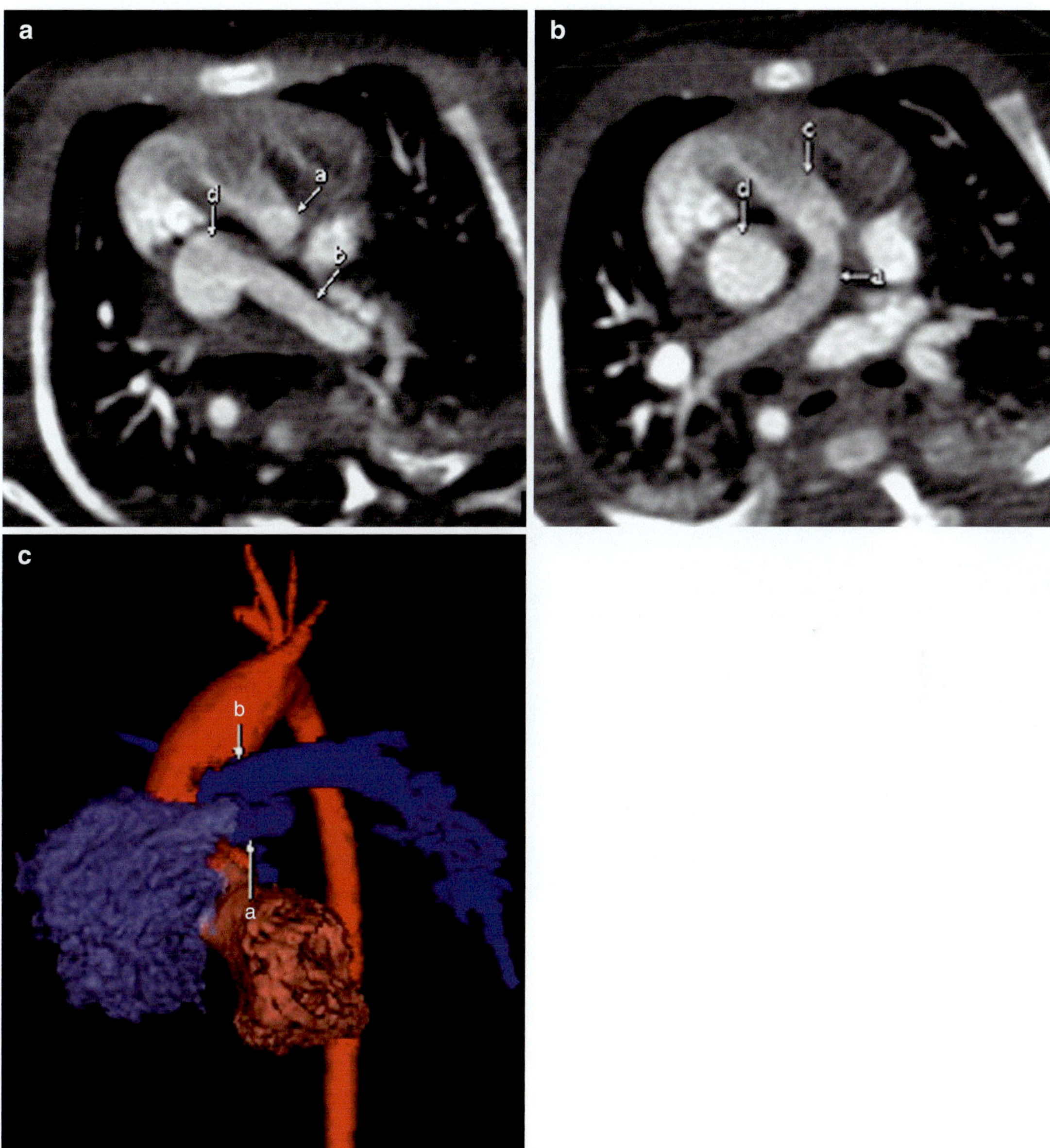

Fig. 7.29 Axial contrast-enhanced (**a b**) and anterior-view color-coded 3D (**c**) images from a cardiac CT scan demonstrating a right ventricular outflow tract (*c*) giving rise to the right pulmonary artery (*a*). The left pulmonary artery (*b*) arises from the ascending aorta (*d*, *red*). This combination is known as a hemitruncus with only half the pulmonary supply coming from the aorta

Pseudotruncus Arteriosus

Pseudotruncus arteriosus is a usually severe form of TOF or pulmonic atresia in which most of the blood flow comes from the aortopulmonary collaterals. In addition to the collaterals, one should look for typical TOF findings: a VSD, right ventricular hypertrophy, an overriding aorta, and pulmonic stenosis.

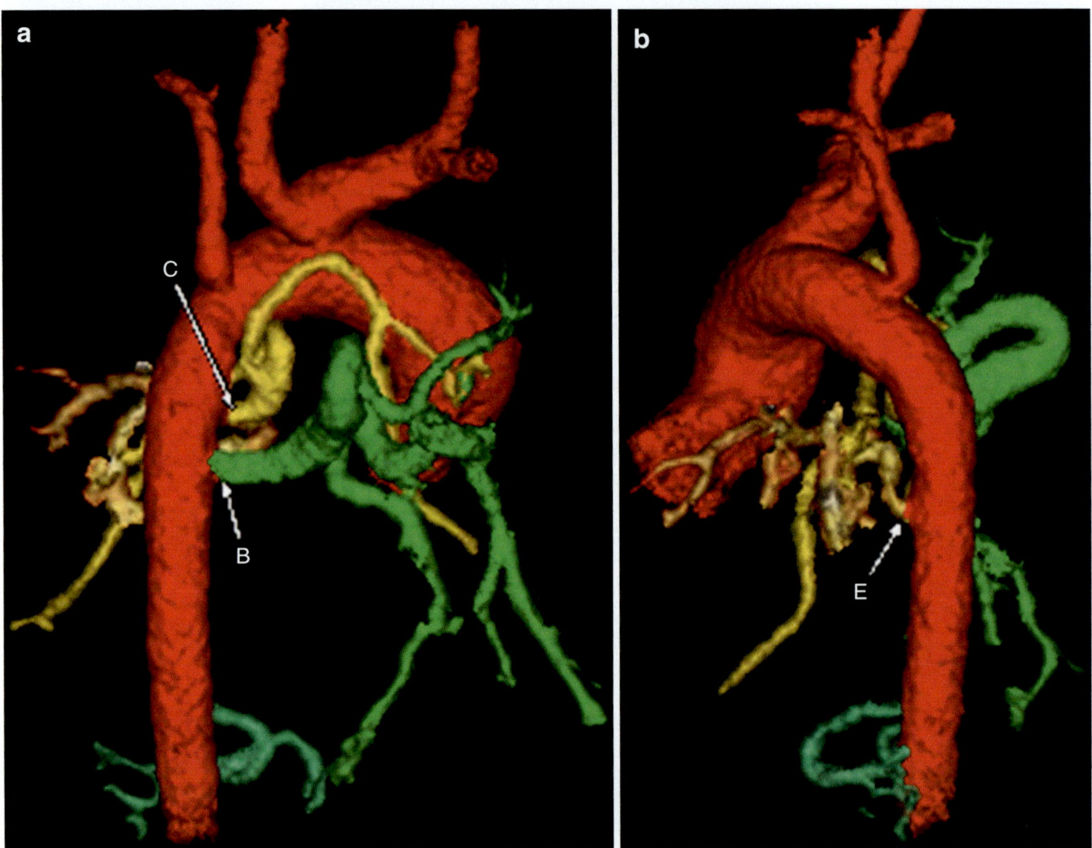

Fig. 7.30 Color-coded 3D (**a** and **b**) and coronal MIP (**c**) images from cardiac CT showing no pulmonary arteries. Instead, all the pulmonary vascular flow is provided by multiple collaterals (*B*, *C*, *E*, and *F*) originating from the descending thoracic aorta

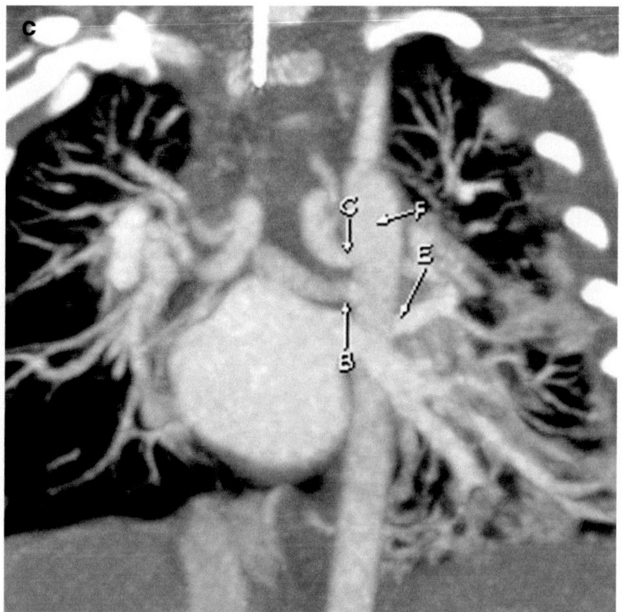

Fig. 7.30 (continued)

Aortopulmonary Window

Aortopulmonary window is the failure of the conotruncal ridges to fuse. Unlike in truncus arteriosus, the pulmonary and aortic valves are normal, with normal proximal aortic and pulmonic outflow tracts. Chest radiography may demonstrate cardiomegaly and increased pulmonary vascularity. A variety of clinical presentations exist depending on the size of the lesion.

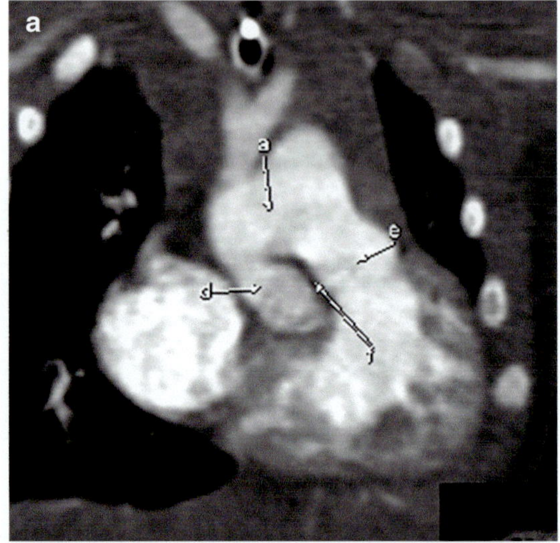

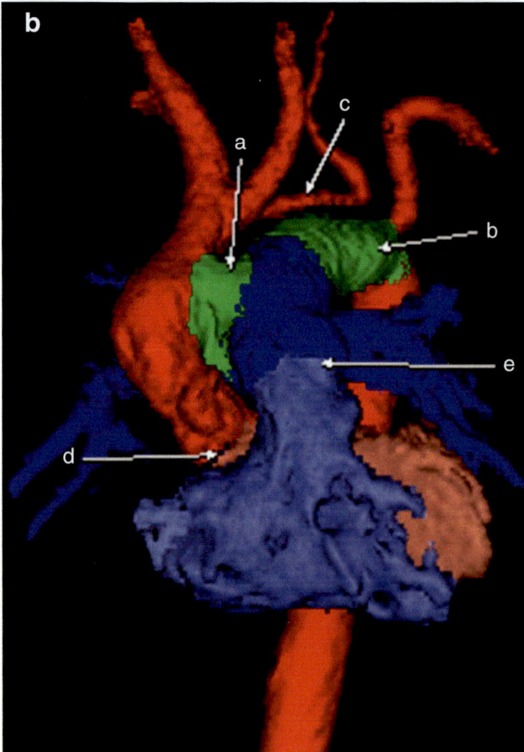

Fig. 7.31 Coronal MIP (**a**) and color-coded 3D (**b**) images from a cardiac CT scan showing an aortopulmonary window lesion (*a*) between the aorta and main pulmonary artery. The pulmonary (*e*) and aortic (*d*) valves are normal in caliber. A PDA (*b*) and an interrupted aortic arch distal to the left common carotid (*c*) also are seen in this case. Notice the normal separation between the pulmonary artery and aorta proximally (*f*)

8 Evaluation of the Coronary Arteries

Randy Ray Richardson and Todd Chapman

The following points should be considered when evaluating the coronary arteries:

1. The origin, number, course, and termination of the coronary arteries should be evaluated. The surgeon should be notified prior to surgery of an anomalous course of the coronaries, especially if it crosses anterior to an outflow tract.
2. The coronary artery rarely may arise from the pulmonary artery, such as in anomalous left coronary artery from the pulmonary artery (ALCAPA).
3. An increased caliber of the coronary arteries in a newborn may suggest a fistulous communication with a low-pressure system, such as the right ventricle, atrium or pulmonary artery.

R.R. Richardson, MD (✉)
Department of Radiology,
St. Joseph's Hospital and Medical Center,
Creighton University School of Medicine,
West Thomas Rd 350, 85013 Phoenix, AZ, USA
e-mail: randy.richardson2@chw.edu,
randy.richardson2@dignityhealth.org

T. Chapman, MD
Radiology Residency Program,
St. Joseph's Hospital and Medical Center,
Phoenix, AZ, USA

R.R. Richardson, *Atlas of Pediatric Cardiac CTA*,
DOI 10.1007/978-1-4614-0088-2_8, © Springer Science+Business Media New York 2013

Normal Coronary Artery Anatomy

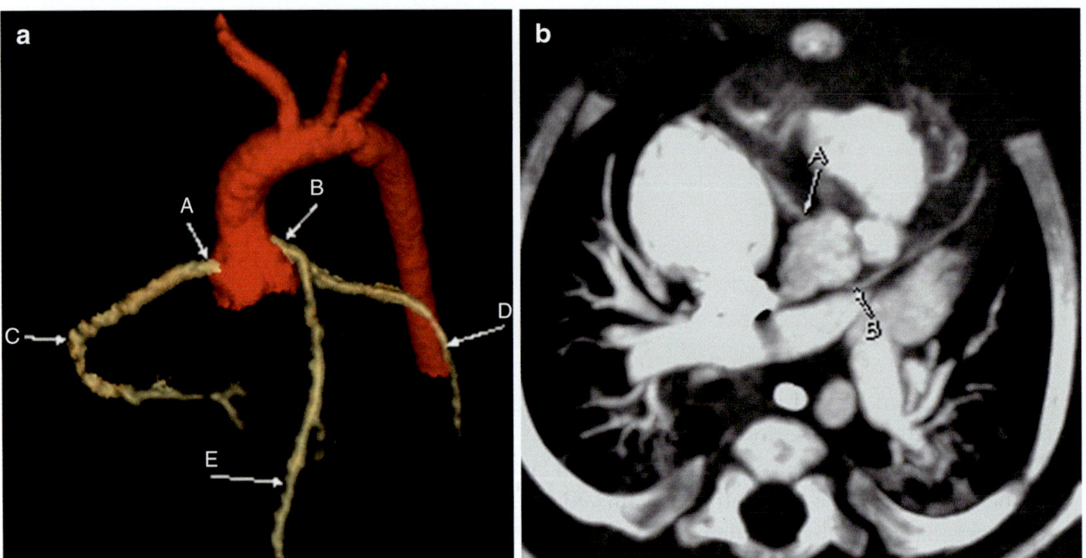

Fig. 8.1 Color-coded three-dimensional (3D; **a**) and axial maximum-intensity projection (MIP; **b**) images from a patient with normal anatomy. The right coronary artery (*C*) arises normally from the right coronary sinus (*A*). The left coronary artery (*B*) arises normally from the left coronary sinus. The left coronary artery divides into the circumflex artery (*D*) and the left anterior descending coronary artery (LAD; *E*)

ALCAPA

ALCAPA (anomalous left coronary artery from the pulmonary artery) is a coronary artery anomaly in which the left coronary artery arises from the pulmonary artery. It leads to cardiac ischemia and infarction, poor left ventricular function, and mitral valve regurgitation. The ischemia typically is a result of a steal phenomenon as the blood is shunted away from the heart to the low-pressure pulmonary artery system through the anomalous coronary artery. Patients with ALCAPA present in infancy with nonspecific symptoms, such as irritability, wheezing, and failure to thrive. The diagnosis usually is made by echocardiography, although cardiac CTA may be used in difficult

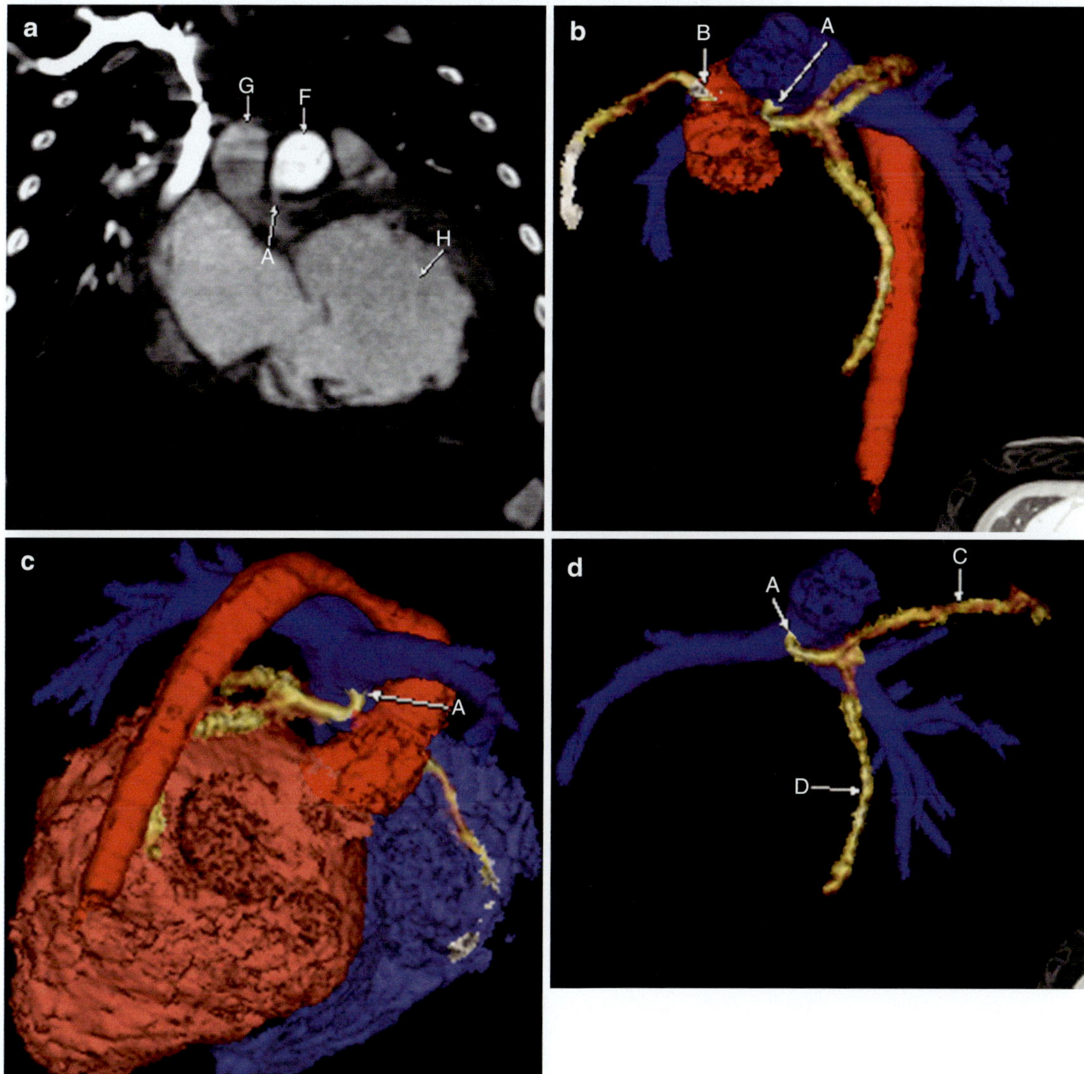

Fig. 8.2 Coronal MIP image (**a**) and color-coded 3D reconstructions (**b–d**) showing the left coronary artery (*A*) arising from the pulmonary artery (*F*, *blue*). The left coronary then branches normally into the LAD (*C*) and circumflex (*D*) arteries. The right coronary artery (*B*) is noted to originate normally from the aorta (*G*, *red*). Notice the dilated left ventricle (*H*)

cases. Findings consist of decreased left ventricular function, an anomalous origin of the coronary artery, and potentially enlarged collateral vessels. ALCAPA may be an isolated finding or may occur with other congenital heart anomalies. Surgical treatment involves either direct transfer of the left coronary artery to the aorta or bypass grafting.

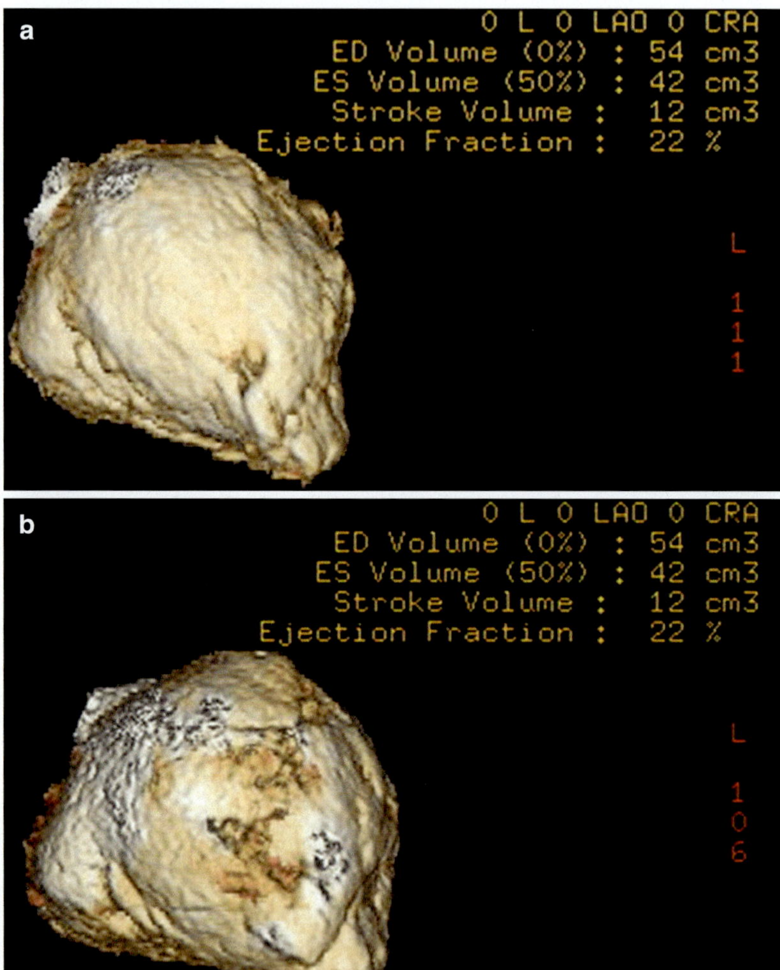

Fig. 8.3 End-systolic (**a**) and end-diastolic (**b**) images from volumetric analysis in a patient with ALCAPA showing a markedly decreased ejection fraction of 22 % and a very dilated left ventricle. The heart failure develops from a steal phenomenon as flow in the anomalous left coronary flows toward the low-pressure pulmonary artery, stealing blood from the heart

Anomalous Right Coronary Artery from the Pulmonary Artery

Anomalous right coronary artery from the pulmonary artery (ARCAPA) is a rare coronary artery origin anomaly in which the right coronary artery arises from the pulmonary artery. As in ALCAPA, patients may present with a variety of nonspecific signs and symptoms, such as heart failure, angina, and myocardial infarction. Cardiac CTA may be used to demonstrate the anomalous origin of the artery. Coronary artery anomalies may be an isolated finding or may be associated with other anomalies. It is important to identify associated defects for surgical planning. Surgical treatment involves either direct transfer of the artery to the aorta or bypass grafting.

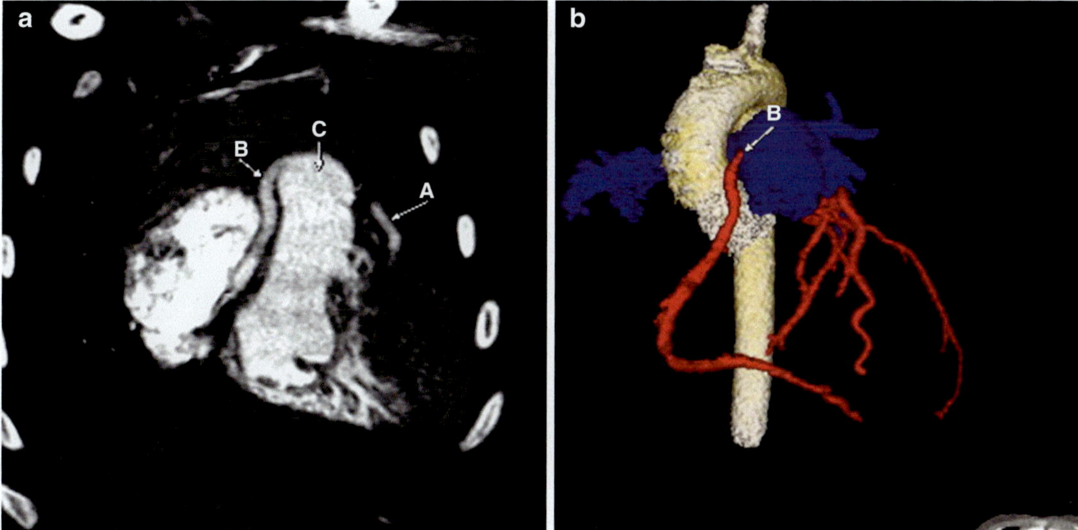

Fig. 8.4 (**a**) Coronal image from a cardiac CTA scan showing the right coronary artery (*B*) arising from the pulmonary artery (*C*). The left coronary artery (*A*), which originates normally from the aorta, also is seen. (**b**) Color-coded 3D model also showing the right coronary artery (*B*) arising from the pulmonary artery (*blue*)

Interarterial (Malignant) Left Coronary Artery

Interarterial left coronary artery is an anomaly in which the left coronary or left anterior descending artery arises from the right sinus of Valsalva (or right coronary artery) and courses between the aorta and the pulmonary artery (interarterial course). Patients are at risk for myocardial ischemia or sudden death with strenuous physical activity. The potential causes of increased morbidity and mortality include coronary artery compression or spasm, a slitlike orifice of the origin of the artery, an acute angle near the ostium, and an intramural course of the proximal artery within the aortic wall. Contrast-enhanced CT is the best imaging modality to evaluate the course of the coronary arteries. Treatment consists of coronary bypass or transfer of the coronary artery to the left sinus of Valsalva.

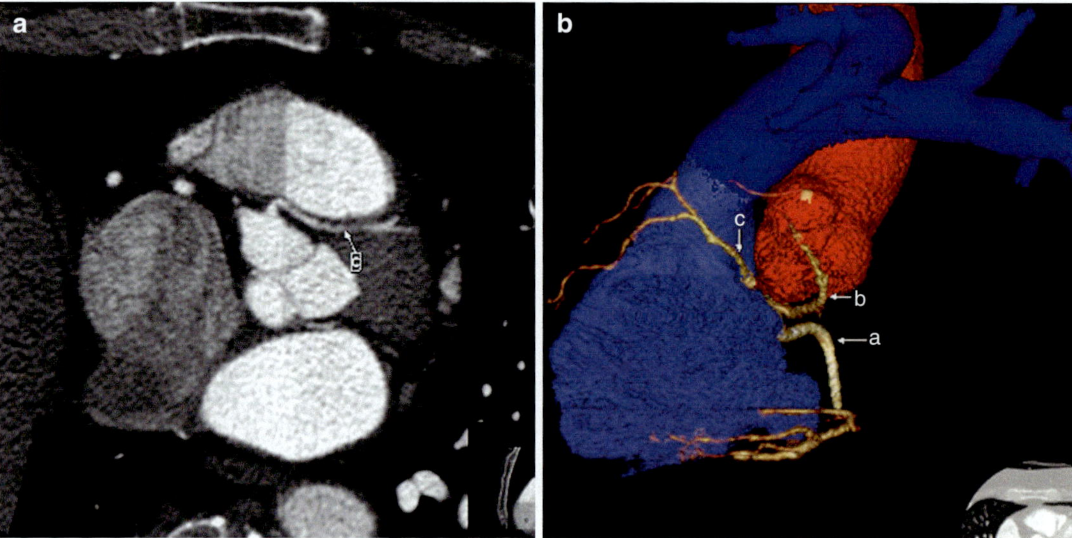

Fig. 8.5 Axial coronary (**a**) and 3D color CTA (**b**) images showing the left anterior descending coronary artery (*c*) arising from the right sinus of Valsalva with an interarterial course between the aorta (*red*) and pulmonary artery (*blue*). The circumflex (*b*) is anomalous, taking a circumaortic course, and arises from the right coronary artery (*a*)

Interarterial (Malignant) Right Coronary Artery

Interarterial right coronary artery is an anomaly in which the right coronary artery arises from the left sinus of Valsalva and courses between the aorta and pulmonary artery. The right coronary artery also may arise from the left main coronary artery or superior to the sinotubular junction. Patients are at risk for sudden death, often precipitated by exercise. The potential causes of increased morbidity and mortality include a slitlike ostium, acute angulation at the origin of the artery, and compression of the vessel between the aorta and pulmonary artery. Cardiac CTA is the best imaging modality to evaluate the coronary anatomy.

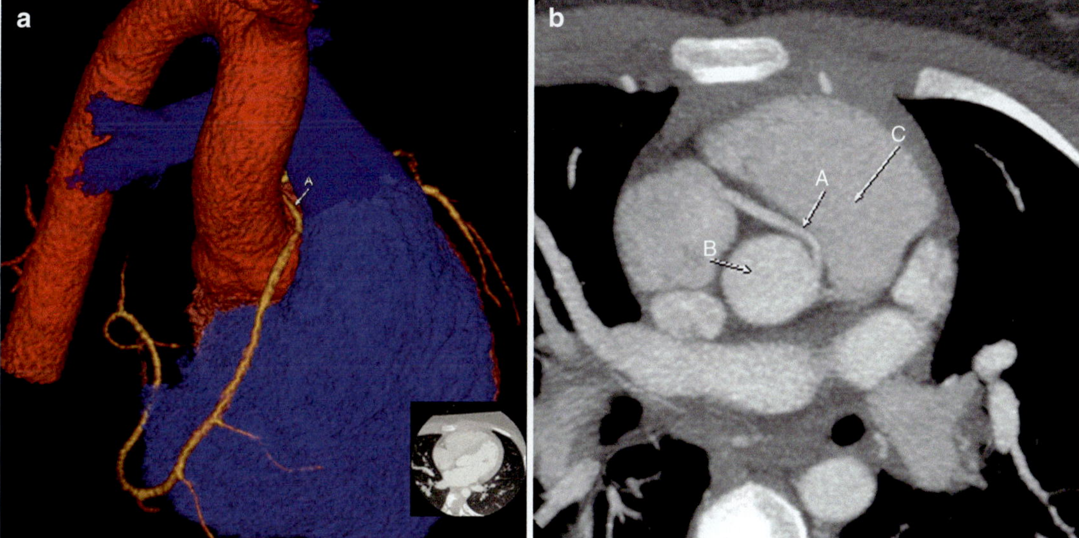

Fig. 8.6 Color-coded 3D (**a**) and axial cardiac CTA (**b**) images demonstrating the right coronary artery (**a**, *A*) arising from the left sinus of Valsalva and coursing between the aorta (*red*, *B*) and pulmonary artery (*blue*). The right ventricle (*C*) is also noted compressing the right coronary artery (*A*)

Prepulmonary Right Coronary Artery

Prepulmonary right coronary artery is an anomaly in which the right coronary artery courses anterior to the pulmonary artery. It is associated with anomalous origin of the right coronary artery, in which the right coronary artery arises from the left sinus of Valsalva or left main coronary artery. It is important to detect this anomaly and alert the surgeon so he or she can avoid severing the vessel during cardiac surgery. This is especially true for patients with tetralogy of Fallot or right ventricular outflow tract stenosis, in which the right coronary artery might be compromised.

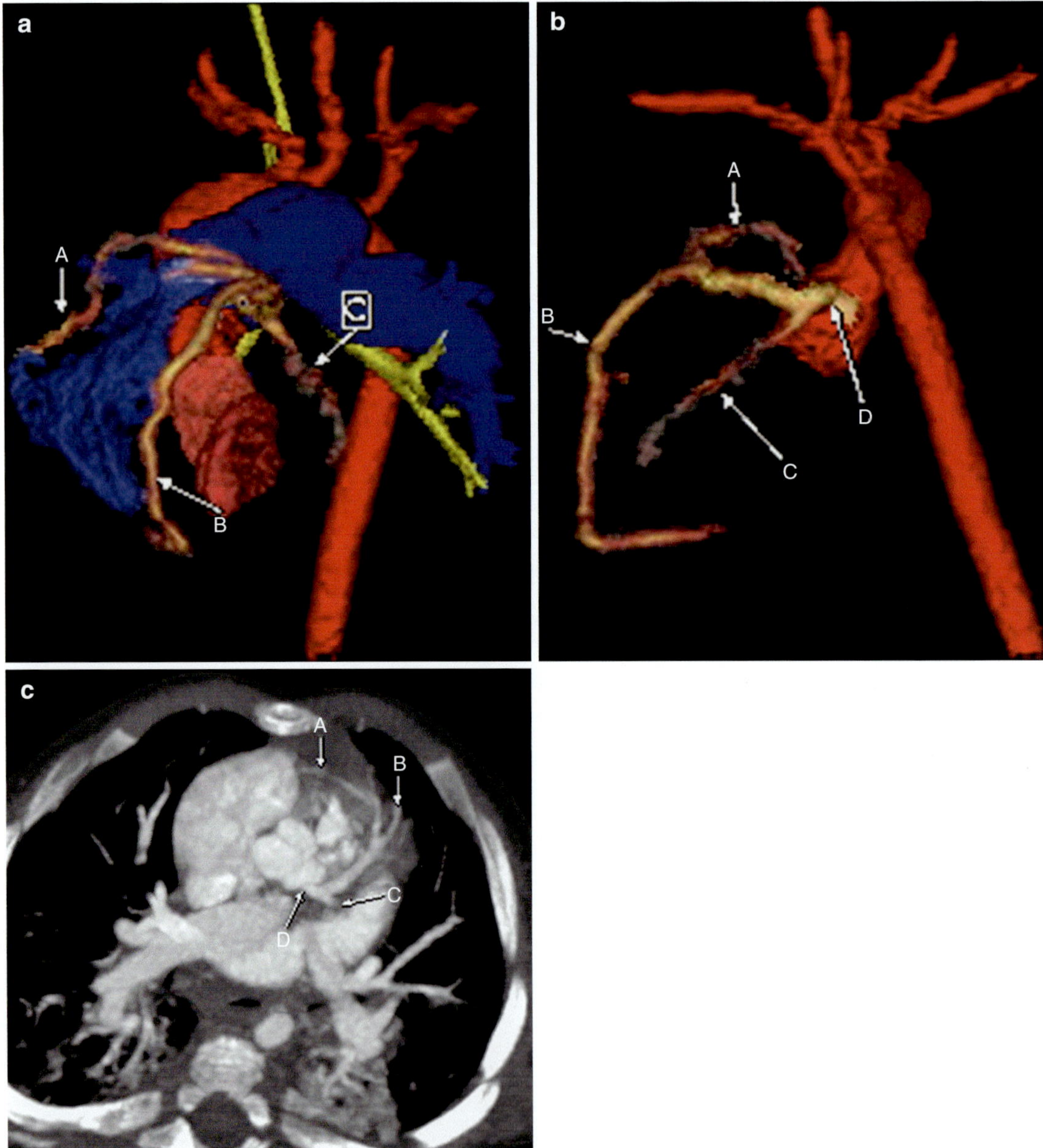

Fig. 8.7 Color-coded 3D reconstructions (**a** and **b**) and axial cardiac CTA scan (**c**) showing the right coronary artery (*A*) arising from the left main coronary artery (*D*) and coursing anterior to the pulmonary artery (*blue*). This position puts the right coronary vessel at risk of being severed during cardiac surgery if the surgeon is not aware of the finding. The left anterior descending (*B*) and left circumflex (*C*) arteries also are noted

Coronary Artery Fistulas

Coronary artery fistulas are abnormal connections between a coronary artery and either a cardiac chamber (coronary cameral fistula) or any portion of the pulmonary or systemic circulation (coronary artery fistula). The coronary artery bypasses the myocardial capillary bed to communicate directly with these structures. The vessel may connect to the pulmonary artery, coronary sinus, atria, or ventricles. Often, there are multiple feeding vessels, which may be tortuous and dilated. Most fistulas are small and cause no symptoms; however, larger fistulas may require surgical intervention.

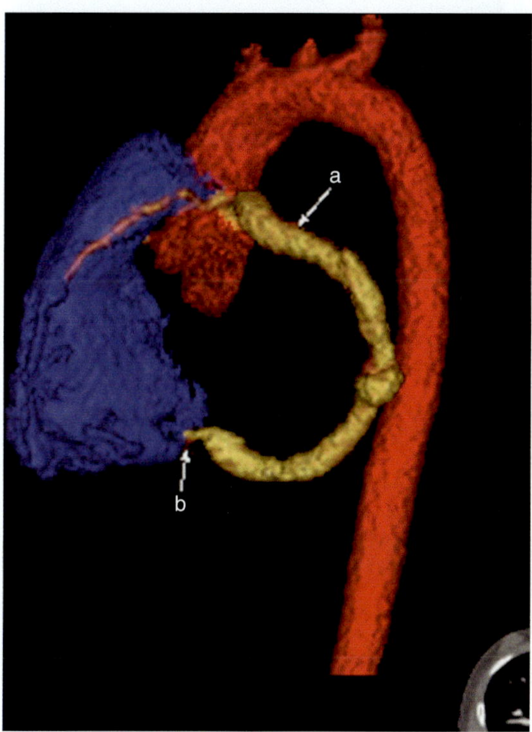

Fig. 8.8 Color-coded 3D reconstruction showing a coronary artery fistula (*b*) between the left coronary artery (*a*) and the right ventricle (*purple*)

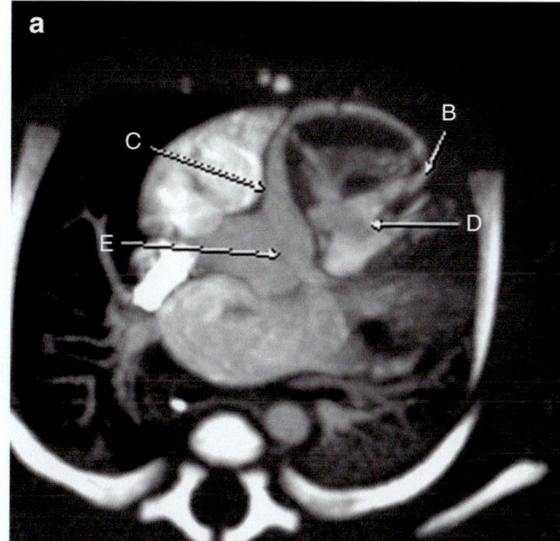

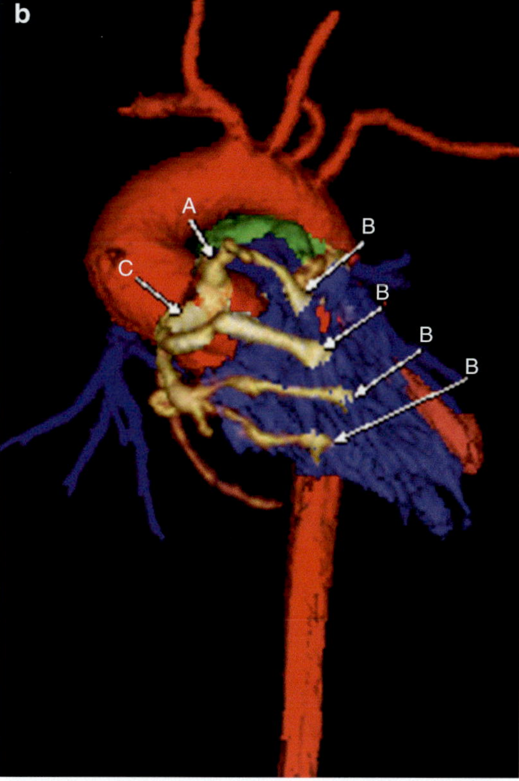

Fig. 8.9 Axial coronary CTA (**a**) and color-coded 3D reconstruction (**b**) images showing the right coronary artery (*C*) arising normally from the aorta (*E*) and forming multiple coronary artery fistulas (*B*) with the right ventricle (*D*, *purple*). A branch of the left coronary artery (*A*) also is noted to be forming a fistula with the right ventricle on the 3D reconstruction

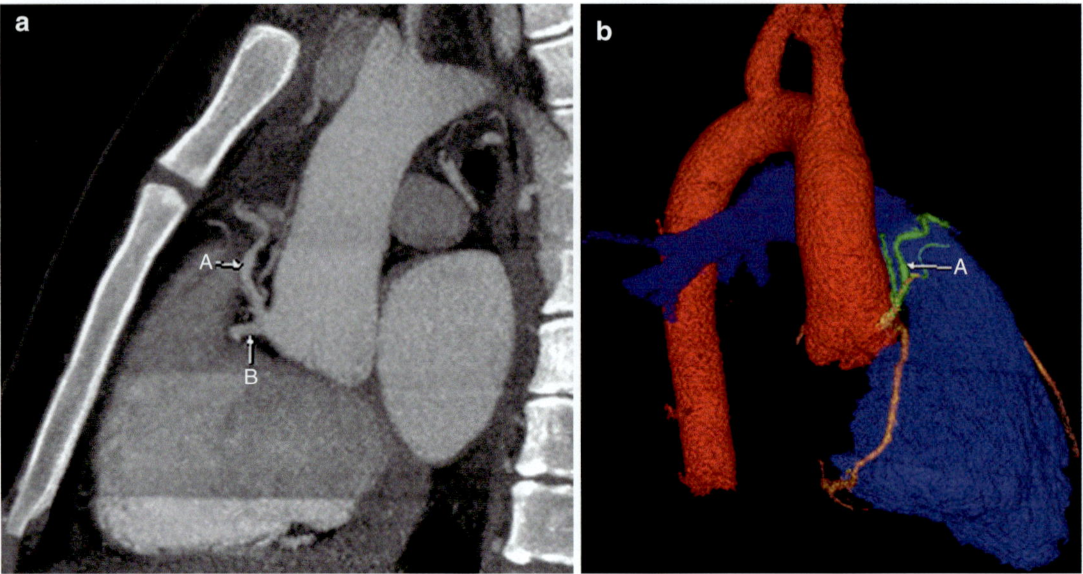

Fig. 8.10 Sagittal coronary CTA image (**a**) and color-coded 3D reconstruction (**b**) showing a branch (*A*, *green*) of the right coronary artery (*B*) forming a fistula with the pulmonary artery (*blue*)

9 Evaluation of the Lungs and Airways

Randy Ray Richardson and Nhi Huynh

The following points should be considered in evaluating the lungs and airways:

1. Congenital airway anomalies are more common in patients with congenital heart disease. Congenital stenosis and bilateral left- or right-sidedness is common in patients with asplenia or polysplenia-type heterotaxies.
2. Specifically, look for a right upper lobe (pig) bronchus, especially in patients with chronic right upper lobe collapse.
3. Tracheobronchomalacia is common in congenital heart disease patients. A narrowed horseshoe-like appearance of the airway may be seen on CT.
4. Extrinsic airway compression is very common in patients with complex congenital heart disease. Look for vascular rings, pulmonary sling, and dilated structures compressing the airway.

R.R. Richardson, MD (✉)
Department of Radiology,
St. Joseph's Hospital and Medical Center,
Creighton University School of Medicine,
West Thomas Rd 350, 85013
Phoenix, AZ, USA
e-mail: randy.richardson2@chw.edu,
randy.richardson2@dignityhealth.org

N. Huynh, MD
Radiology Residency Program,
St. Joseph's Hospital and Medical Center,
Phoenix, AZ, USA

Normal Anatomy

Normally, the right mainstem bronchus courses posterior and slightly superior to the right main pulmonary artery (eparterial bronchus), with the right upper lobe bronchus arising more proximal than the left. The left mainstem bronchus courses under the left main pulmonary artery (hyparterial bronchus).

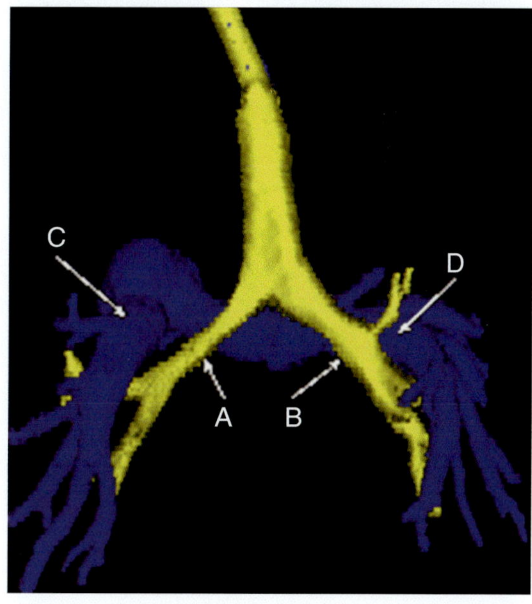

Fig. 9.1 Posterior projection from a cardiac CTA image showing a typical left bronchus (*A*), which is elongated and is known as a hyparterial bronchus because the left main pulmonary artery (*C*) is draped over the proximal left bronchus (*A*). The right main bronchus (*B*) has a shorter course before giving off the upper lobe bronchus more proximally. Notice that the left main pulmonary artery (*D*) is not draped over the bronchus (*B*). This is known as an *eparterial bronchus*

R.R. Richardson, *Atlas of Pediatric Cardiac CTA*,
DOI 10.1007/978-1-4614-0088-2_9, © Springer Science+Business Media New York 2013

Tracheal (Pig) Bronchus

A tracheal, or pig, bronchus is an anatomic variant (typically right) upper lobe bronchus originating from the trachea above the carina. Two types exist: displaced bronchus and supernumerary bronchus. This condition may cause persistent or recurrent right upper lobe pneumonias.

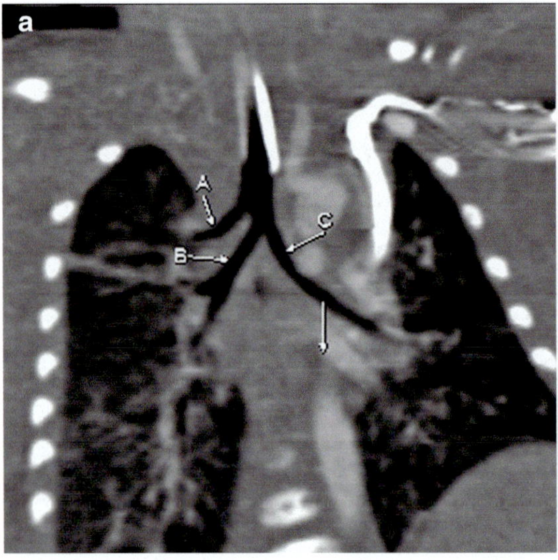

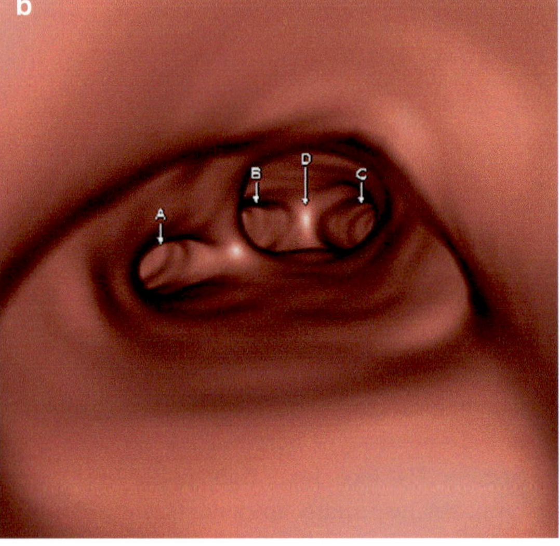

Fig. 9.2 Coronal (**a**) and virtual bronchoscopy. Descending aorta (*arrow*) is shown. (**b**) Images demonstrating a right upper lobe accessory bronchus (*A*) arising from the trachea above the carina (*D*). The right bronchus (*B*) and left main bronchus (*C*) are shown

Airway Compression from Enlarged Pulmonary Arteries

Enlarged pulmonary arteries, when present, may be a frequent cause of airway compression in infants and small children with congenital heart disease. Enlarged pulmonary arteries frequently are seen in patients with congenital absence of the pulmonic valve, as observed in tetralogy of Fallot variants.

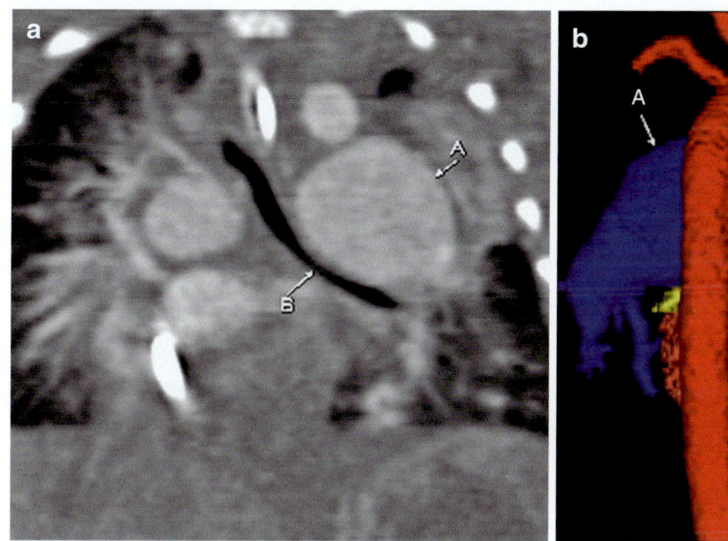

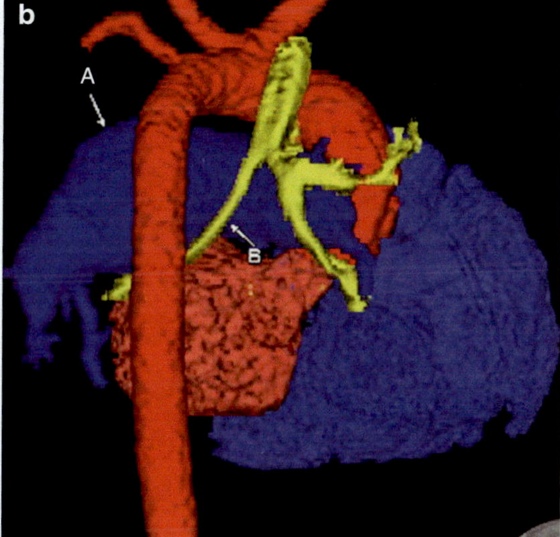

Fig. 9.3 Enhanced coronal (**a**) and posterior projection color-coded three-dimensional (3D; **b**) images showing an enlarged left main pulmonary artery (*A*) with mass effect, resulting in moderate narrowing of the adjacent left main bronchus (*B*)

Tracheobronchomalacia

Tracheobronchomalacia is a tracheobronchial cartilaginous abnormality resulting in abnormally increased pliability and intermittent airway collapse. Dynamic examination, such as fluoroscopy or endoscopy, shows characteristic changes in airway caliber. Tracheobronchomalacia may be primary or secondary.

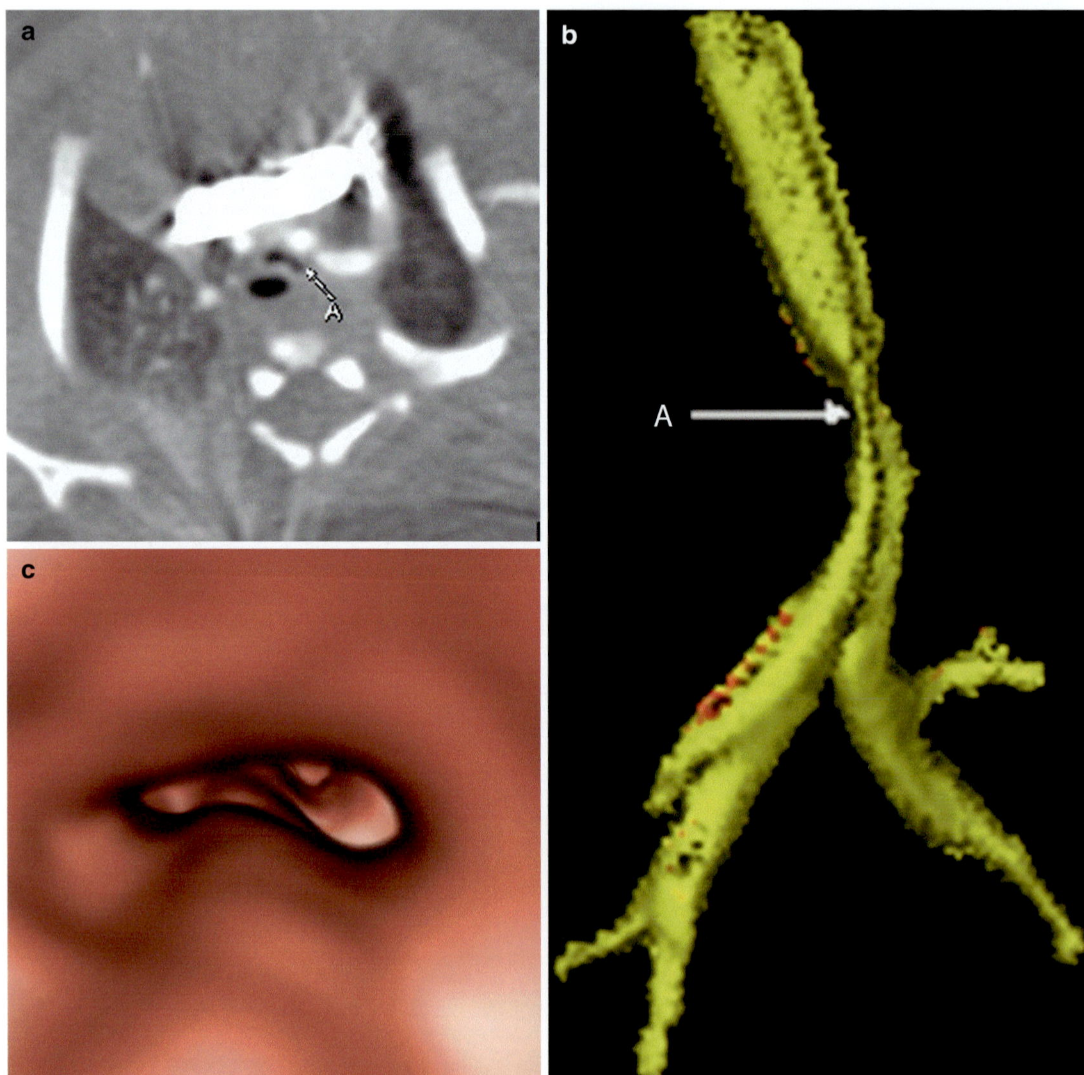

Fig. 9.4 Enhanced axial (**a**), lateral projection color-coded 3D (**b**), and virtual bronchoscopy (**c**) images show an area of mid-tracheal narrowing (*A*) consistent with tracheomalacia. Notice the characteristic horseshoe shape of the trachea (*A*) which is a typical CT finding in patients with tracheomalacia

Double Aortic Arch

Double aortic arch is the congenital persistence of both left and right fourth embryologic arches. Two arches surround and compress the trachea anteriorly and esophagus posteriorly. Surgical management is altered depending on whether the right or left arch is dominant; the right arch more commonly is dominant. Double aortic arch is the most common symptomatic vascular anomaly. It forms a true vascular ring.

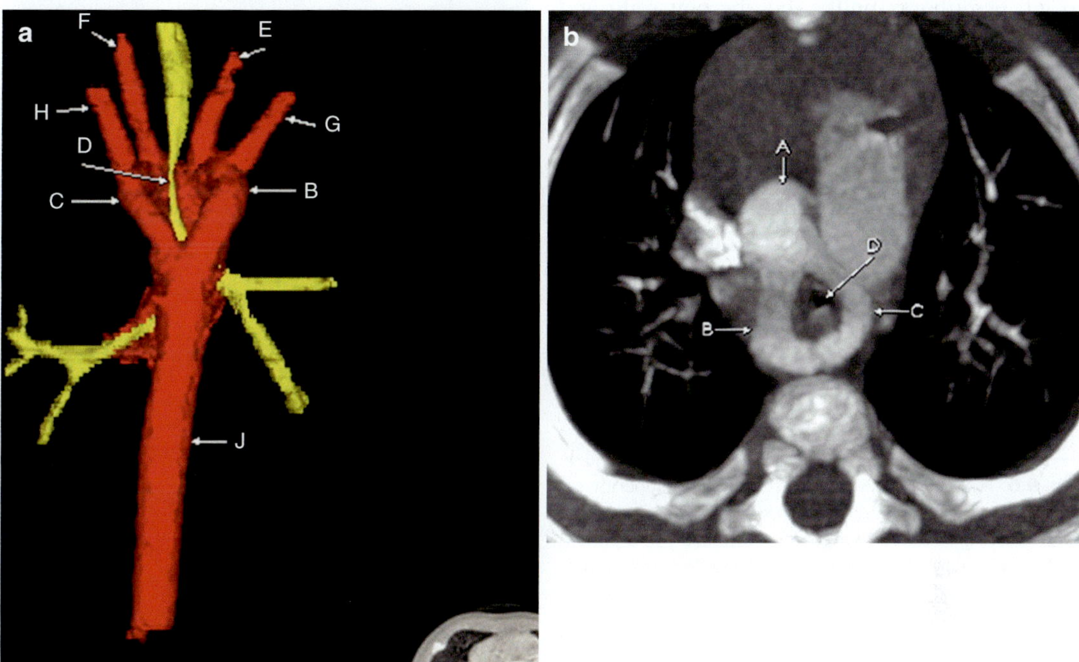

Fig. 9.5 Posterior projection color-coded 3D (**a**) and enhanced axial CT (**b**) images showing tracheal compression (*D*) by the surrounding vascular ring formed by the right (*B*) and left (*C*) aortic arches, which divide from the ascending aorta (*A*) and join again posteriorly to form the descending aorta (*J*). There is symmetric branching of the great vessels, with the right (*E*) and left (*F*) carotid and right (*G*) and left (*H*) subclavian arteries arising from the corresponding aortic arch.

Pulmonary Sling

Pulmonary sling is an anomaly in which the left pulmonary artery originates from the right pulmonary artery and then courses around the trachea and proximal mainstem bronchi, often resulting in severe airway compression. The anomalous left pulmonary artery courses between the trachea and esophagus as it crosses from the right to left hemithorax unlike the aberrant right and left subclavian arteries, which typically course posterior to the esophagus. Airway compression often is asymmetric and may result in unilateral hyperinflation from air trapping. On a lateral esophagram, indentation of the posterior trachea and anterior esophagus is characteristic. Pulmonary sling is not a true vascular ring.

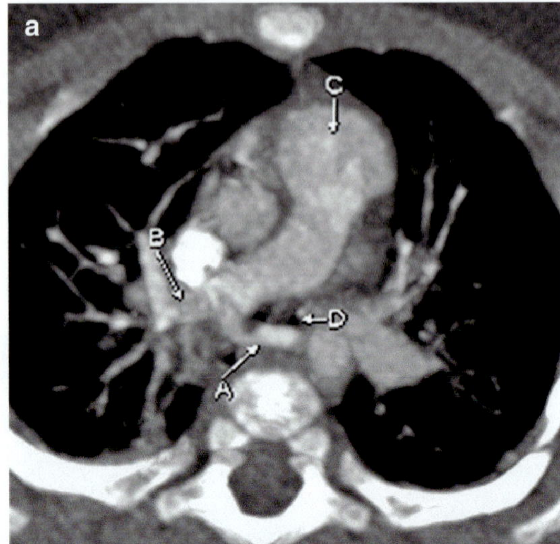

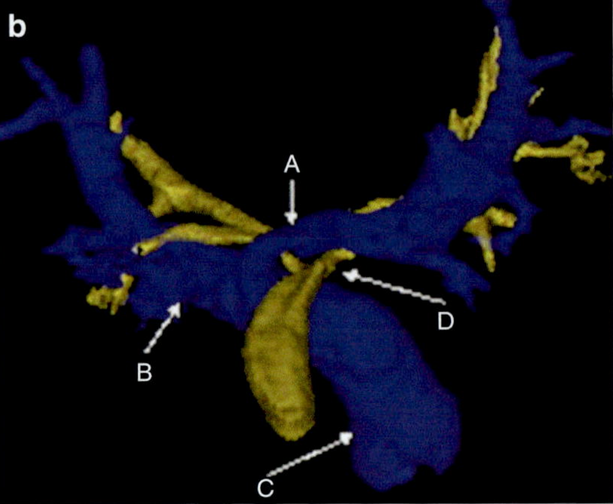

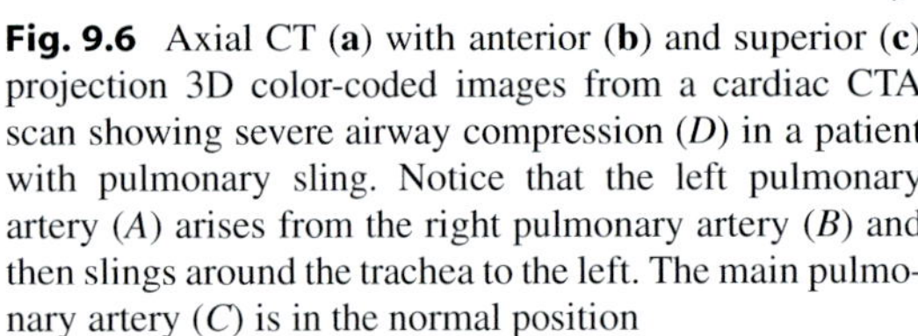

Fig. 9.6 Axial CT (**a**) with anterior (**b**) and superior (**c**) projection 3D color-coded images from a cardiac CTA scan showing severe airway compression (*D*) in a patient with pulmonary sling. Notice that the left pulmonary artery (*A*) arises from the right pulmonary artery (*B*) and then slings around the trachea to the left. The main pulmonary artery (*C*) is in the normal position

Right Aortic Arch with Aberrant Left Subclavian Artery

Right aortic arch with an aberrant left subclavian artery (RAA-ALSCA) is a true vascular ring when the patent ductus arteriosus (PDA) arises from the aberrant right subclavian artery. In this scenario, the right arch (right), aberrant subclavian (posterior), pulmonary artery (anterior), and PDA (left) form a complete vascular ring around the trachea and esophagus. Tracheal narrowing and stridor are common, but the patient may become increasingly symptomatic with time.

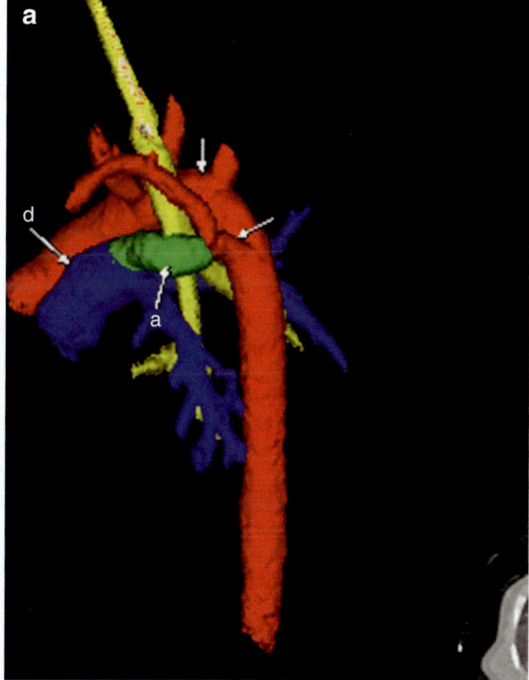

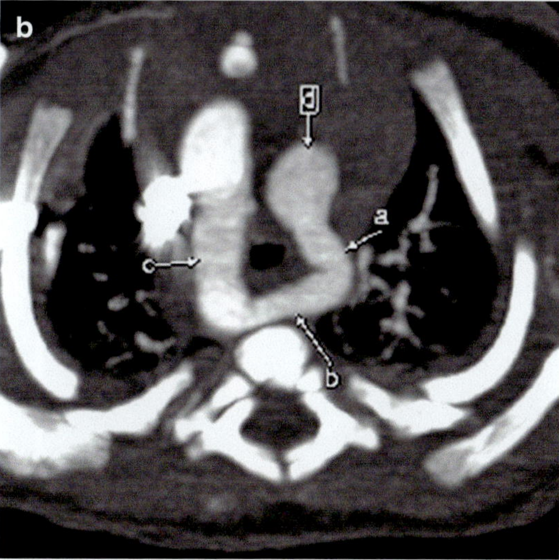

Fig. 9.7 Color-coded 3D (**a**) and axial CT (**b**) images from a cardiac CTA scan showing a right aortic arch (*c*) with an aberrant left subclavian artery (*b*). The PDA (*a*) arising from the main pulmonary artery (*d*) completes the vascular ring around the trachea (*yellow*) and esophagus

Right Aortic Arch with Aberrant Left Subclavian Artery with Kommerell Diverticulum

RAA-ALSCA often occurs with a Kommerell diverticulum, which is seen as a focal dilatation at the origin of the aberrant subclavian artery off the descending right aortic arch. A Kommerell diverticulum may be present in patients with a left aortic arch and an aberrant right subclavian artery but is much less common.

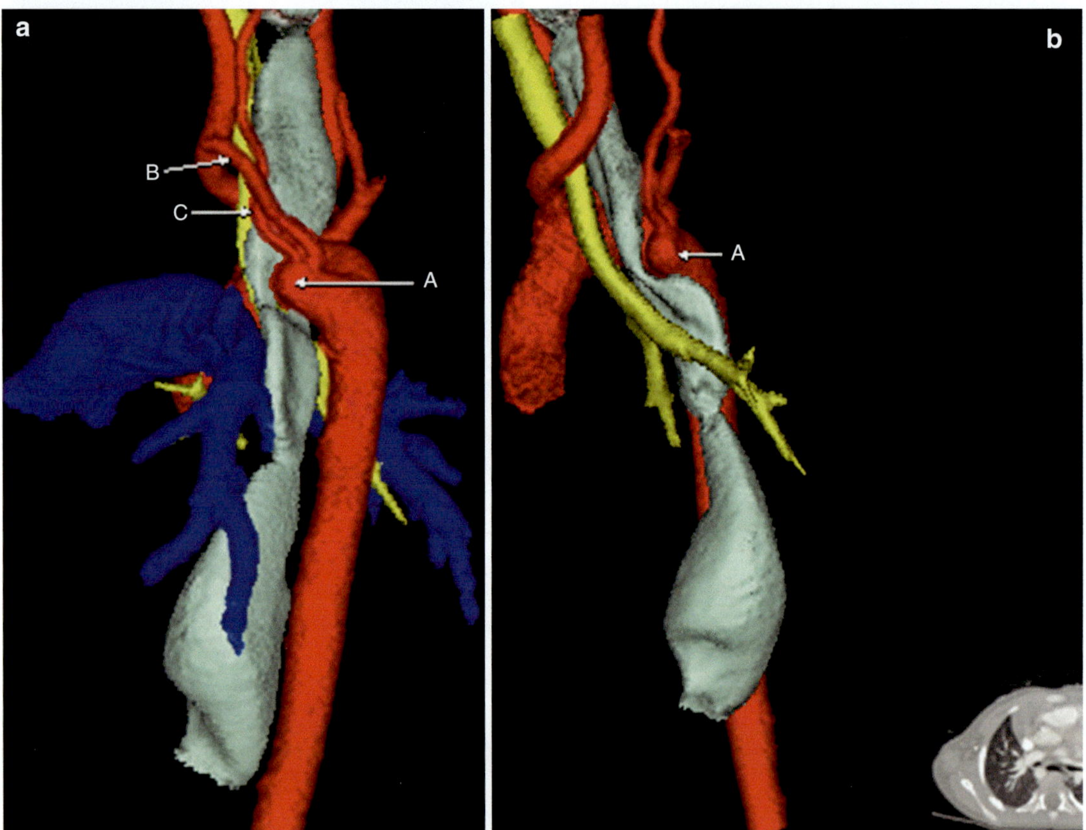

Fig. 9.8 (**a**, **b**) Color-coded 3D images from a cardiac CTA scan showing mild airway compression in a patient with a right arch and aberrant left subclavian (*B*) and vertebral (*C*) arteries. Notice the compression of the esophagus (*green*) and the contouring of the trachea (*yellow*) from the large diverticulum of Kommerell (*A*)

10 Evaluation of Situs

Randy Ray Richardson and Nhi Huynh

In evaluating situs, the following points should be considered:

1. Each patient should be designated as situs solitus (normal), situs inversus (reversed), or situs ambiguous (indeterminate).
2. Situs usually is determined by the sidedness of the liver, stomach, spleen, right atrial appendages, inferior vena cava (IVC) and cardiac position. In addition, the anatomy of the tracheobronchial tree and the relationship of the right and left mainstem bronchi with respect to the right and left pulmonary arteries are important hallmarks.
3. The normal heart is in levocardia (at the left chest) and with the apex pointed to the left. Dextrocardia occurs when the heart is in the right side of the chest. Here, the apex may be pointed to the right or to the left. Mesocardia is the condition in which the heart is in the midline and the apex is pointed inferiorly or is difficult to ascertain.
4. When structures above are normally positioned, it is termed *situs solitus*. When the structures are reversed, it is termed *situs inversus*. When there is a combination of both, it typically is termed *situs ambiguous*.
5. The presence of situs ambiguous may be a hallmark of asplenia and polysplenia heterotaxy syndrome.

R.R. Richardson, MD (✉)
Department of Radiology,
St. Joseph's Hospital and Medical Center,
Creighton University School of Medicine,
West Thomas Rd 350, 85013 Phoenix, AZ, USA
e-mail: randy.richardson2@chw.edu,
randy.richardson2@dignityhealth.org

N. Huynh, MD
Radiology Residency Program,
St. Joseph's Hospital and Medical Center,
Phoenix, AZ, USA

R.R. Richardson, *Atlas of Pediatric Cardiac CTA*,
DOI 10.1007/978-1-4614-0088-2_10,

Normal Anatomy (Situs Solitus)

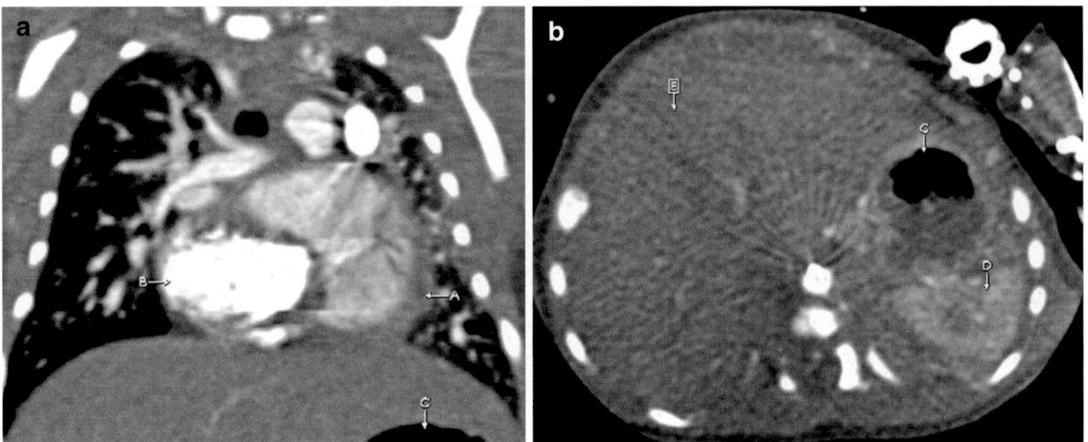

Fig. 10.1 Coronal (**a**) and axial (**b**) images from a cardiac CTA scan showing the spleen (*D*) and stomach (*C*) on the left, with the apex of the heart (*A*) on the left and the right atrium (*B*) on the right. The liver (*E*) is on the right. These findings are consistent with situs solitus

Polysplenia Syndrome–Type Heterotaxy

Patients with polysplenia syndrome–type heterotaxy have polysplenia; anomalous pulmonary venous return, which often is partial instead of complete; bilateral superior vena cava (SVC); left isomerism of the atrial appendages; bilateral hyparterial bronchi with bilateral bilobed lungs; and azygous continuation of the IVC.

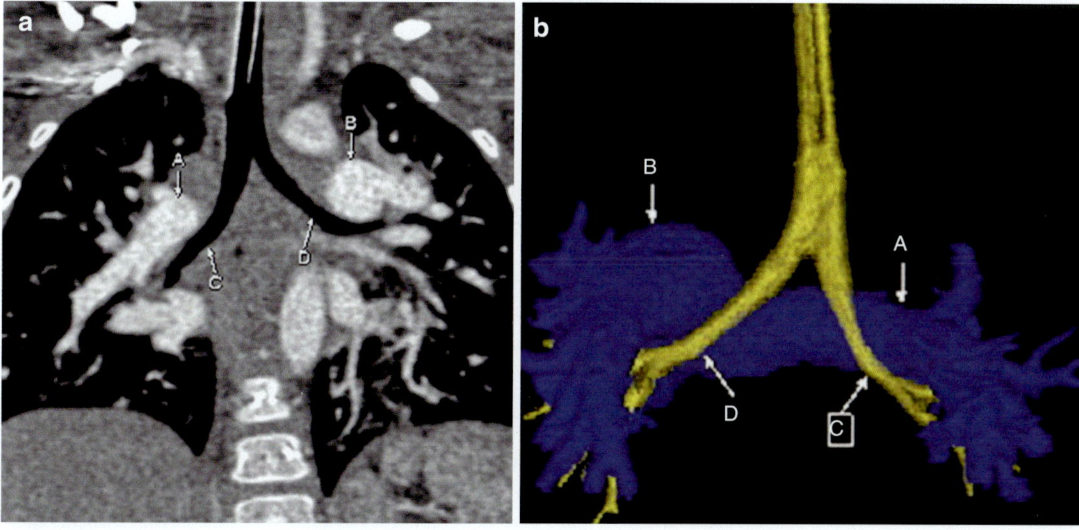

Fig. 10.2 Enhanced coronal (**a**) and posterior projection color-coded three-dimensional (3D; **b**) images showing that the right (*C*) and left (*D*) bronchi are inferior to the right (*A*) and left (*B*) pulmonary arteries, respectively. These findings are compatible with bilateral left-sided tracheobronchial branching (bilateral hyparterial bronchi) in a patient with a polysplenia heterotaxy. Notice that both bronchi (*C* and *D*) are elongated, consistent with left-sided bronchial morphology

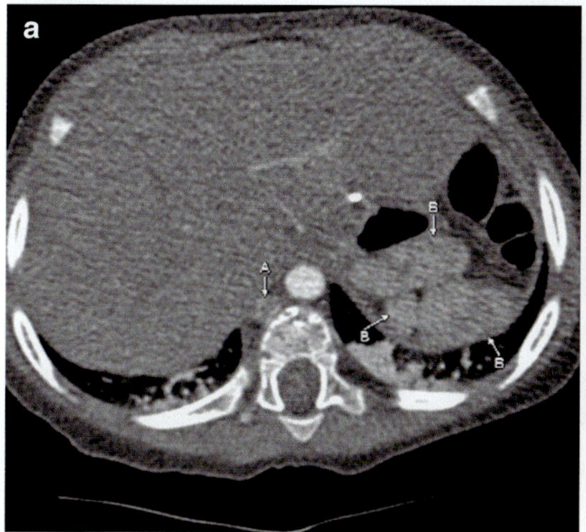

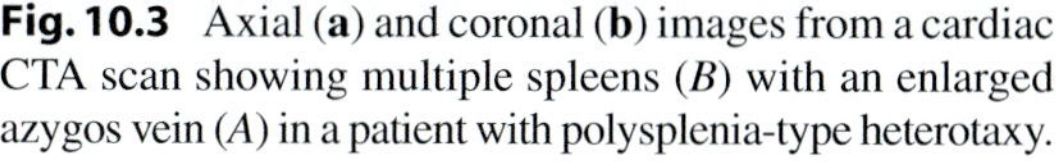
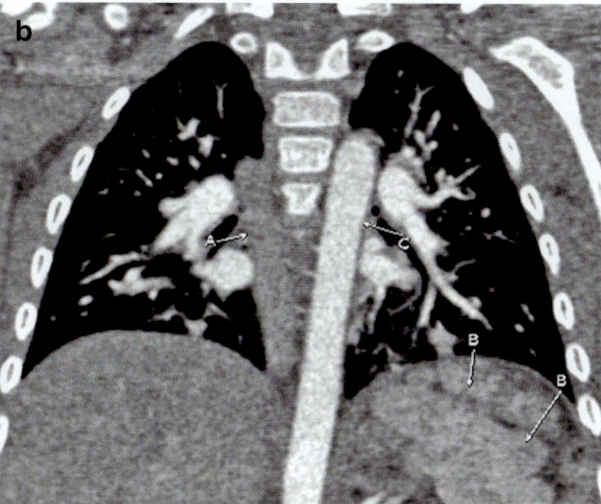

Fig. 10.3 Axial (**a**) and coronal (**b**) images from a cardiac CTA scan showing multiple spleens (*B*) with an enlarged azygos vein (*A*) in a patient with polysplenia-type heterotaxy. Notice that the descending aorta (*C*) is to the left of the enlarged azygos vein

Asplenia Syndrome–Type Heterotaxy

Asplenia syndrome–type heterotaxy often consists of a bilateral SVC, right isomerism of the atrial appendages, bilateral right-sided tracheobronchial branching, and anomalous pulmonary venous connections with complex congenital heart disease.

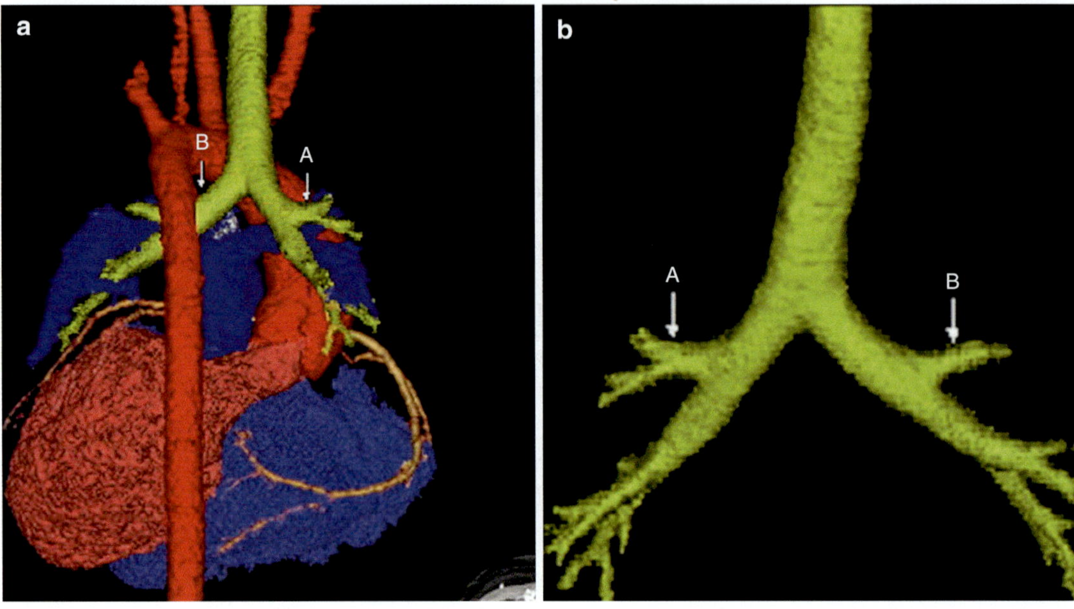

Fig. 10.4 Posterior (**a**) and anterior (**b**) color-coded 3D images from a cardiac CTA scan showing symmetric bilateral right-sided bronchi (*A* and *B*), with the bronchi arising above the level of the right and left main pulmonary arteries (*blue*) and early branching of the mainstem bronchi (*A* and *B*), which is typical right bronchial morphology. These findings are seen with bilateral right-sided tracheobronchial (bilateral eparterial bronchi) branching

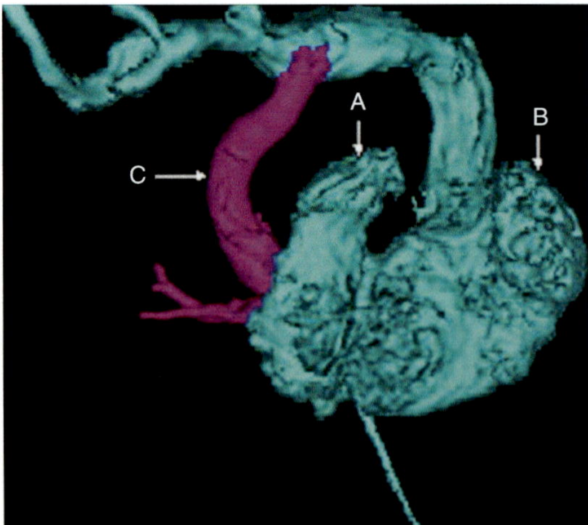

Fig. 10.5 Frontal color-coded image from a cardiac CTA scan showing symmetric bilateral right atria (*light blue*) with very symmetric-appearing atrial appendages (*A* and *B*). Because there is no left atrium, the pulmonary veins often take an anomalous route back to the heart, as seen in this case with an anomalous vertical vein (*C*) draining the pulmonary veins (*pink*) superiorly to the brachiocephalic vein (*light blue*)

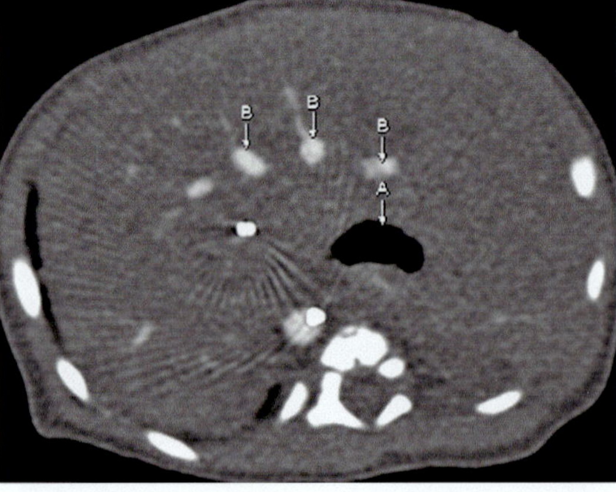

Fig. 10.6 Axial image from a cardiac CTA scan showing a midline liver with symmetric draining hepatic veins (*B*). Notice the midline stomach (*A*) and the absence of a spleen in this patient with asplenia-type heterotaxy

Complex Congenital Heart Disease in a Patient with Asplenia-Type Heterotaxy

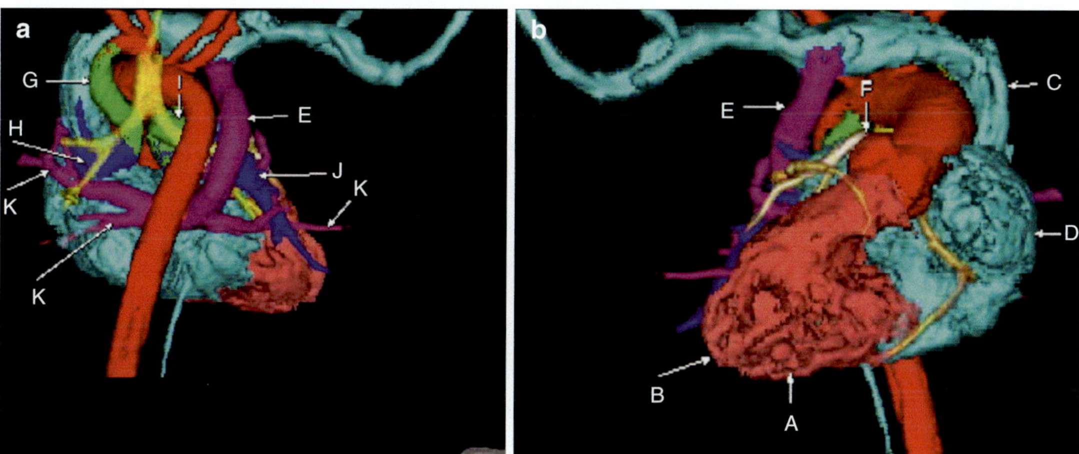

Fig. 10.7 Frontal (**a**) and posterior (**b**) projection images from a cardiac CTA scan showing a patient with asplenia-type heterotaxy. There is situs inversus with the apex of the heart (*B*) on the right, a large common atrium (*D*), and the SVC (*C*) on the left. Complex congenital heart disease is shown with a common ventricle (*A*) and the aorta (*F*, *red*) as the only outflow tract from the heart. The pulmonary arteries (*H* and *J*) arise from a bilateral patent ductus arteriosus (PDA; *G* and *I*). The left PDA (*G*), gives rise to the left pulmonary artery (*H*) and the right PDA (*I*) on the right (*I*) that supplies the right pulmonary artery (*J*). There is total anomalous pulmonary venous return with the pulmonary veins (*K*) draining to an anomalous vertical vein (*E*), which empties superiorly into the brachiocephalic vein (*light blue*)

11 Operations Performed for Patients with Congenital Heart Disease

Randy Ray Richardson and Nhi Huynh

When dealing with congenital heart disease, it is vital to understand the basic terminology regarding postoperative shunts, procedures, and surgeries.

Sano Shunt

A Sano shunt is a vascular conduit that shunts blood from the right ventricle to the main pulmonary artery. The shunt narrows as it traverses the right ventricular wall, which limits regurgitant flow. It may be used in combination with a Blalock-Taussig (BT) shunt in patients with hypoplastic left heart syndrome as part I of the Norwood procedure.

R.R. Richardson, MD (✉)
Department of Radiology,
St. Joseph's Hospital and Medical Center,
Creighton University School of Medicine,
West Thomas Rd 350, 85013 Phoenix, AZ, USA
e-mail: randy.richardson2@chw.edu,
randy.richardson2@dignityhealth.org

N. Huynh, MD
Radiology Residency Program,
St. Joseph's Hospital and Medical Center,
Phoenix, AZ, USA

R.R. Richardson, *Atlas of Pediatric Cardiac CTA*,
DOI 10.1007/978-1-4614-0088-2_11, © Springer Science+Business Media New York 2013

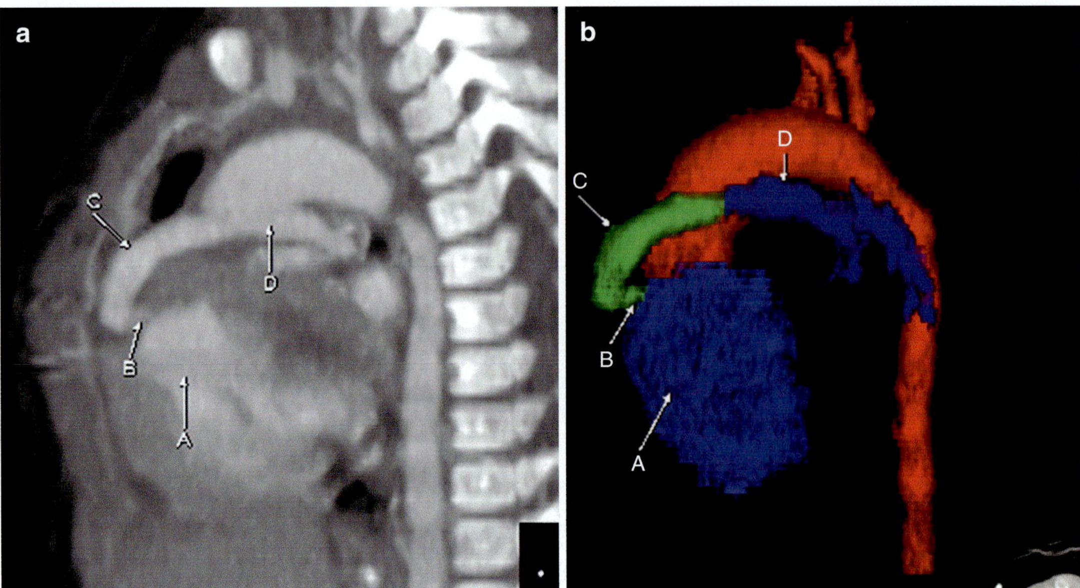

Fig. 11.1 Sagittal maximum-intensity projection (MIP; **a**) and color-coded three-dimensional (3D; **b**) images showing a Sano shunt (*C*) connecting the right ventricle (*A*) to the main pulmonary artery (*D*). Notice the stenotic portion of the proximal shunt (*B*), where the conduit traverses the right ventricular wall

Modified BT Shunt

The modified BT shunt uses a vascular graft (typically Gore-Tex [W. L. Gore and Associates, Elkton, MD]) that shunts blood from the subclavian or brachiocephalic artery to the ipsilateral main pulmonary artery. It often is used as a palliative procedure to increase pulmonary flow and expand the pulmonary arteries before more definitive surgery. The modified shunt differs from the original procedure, which is performed without a graft.

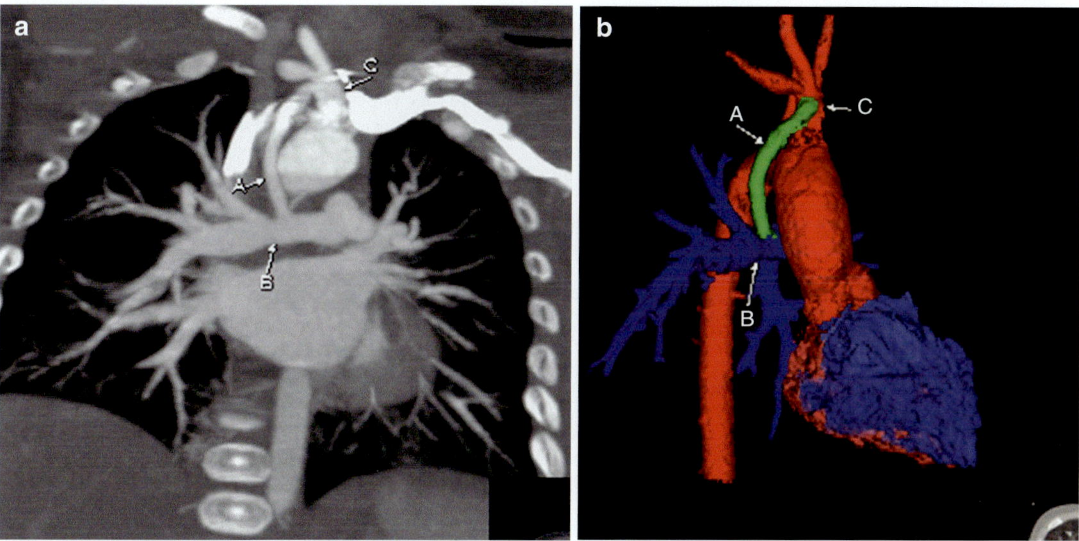

Fig. 11.2 Enhanced coronal (**a**) and color-coded 3D (**b**) images showing a modified BT shunt (*A*) connecting the right brachiocephalic artery (*C*) to the right main pulmonary artery (*B*)

Glenn Shunt

The Glenn shunt is a vascular conduit that shunts blood from the superior vena cava (SVC) to the right pulmonary artery. It is used in a staged palliative procedure in patients with single-ventricle physiology. Eventually, a more definitive Fontan shunt is performed to also supply blood from the inferior vena cava (IVC) to the pulmonary arteries. Glenn shunts typically are performed at 3–9 months of age, when pulmonary vascular resistance has decreased. If a left SVC also is present, bilateral bidirectional Glenn shunts are performed.

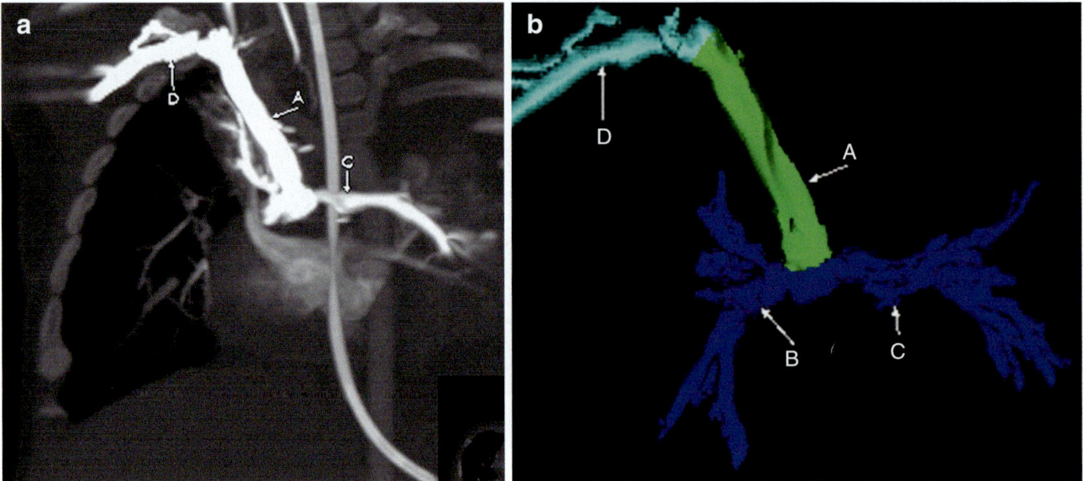

Fig. 11.3 Coronal MIP (**a**) and color-coded 3D (**b**) images showing a Glenn shunt channeling upper-extremity blood flow from the SVC (*A*) to the right pulmonary artery (*B*). The flow is bidirectional, with the left pulmonary artery (*C*) also filling. Contrast was injected from the right upper extremity, with the right subclavian vein (*D*) also opacified

Fontan Procedure

The Fontan procedure involves the placement of a vascular shunt that channels blood from the IVC to the pulmonary artery. It is the final procedure for patients with single-ventricle physiology to provide definitive blood flow to the pulmonary arteries. The surgery may be intra-atrial, in which a tunnel is created to channel blood to the pulmonary arteries, or extra-atrial in which a synthetic graft is placed to connect the IVC to the pulmonary arteries.

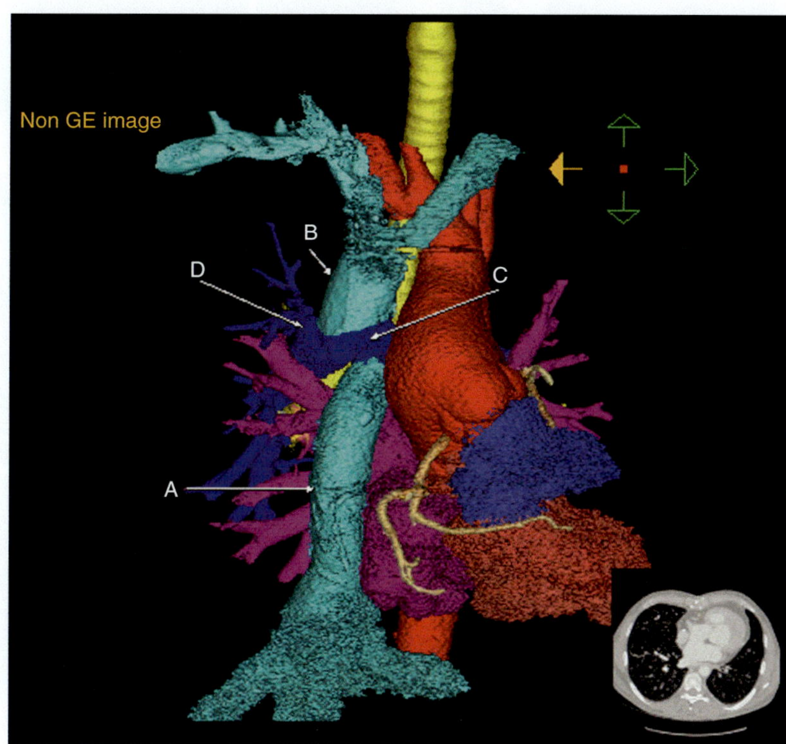

Fig. 11.4 Color-coded 3D image from a CTA scan showing an extracardiac Fontan graft (*A*) extending from the IVC to the main pulmonary artery (*C*). Also notice the presence of a Glenn shunt (*B*) channeling blood from the SVC to the right main pulmonary artery (*D*)

Hybrid Procedure

The hybrid procedure typically is performed for palliation in patients with hypoplastic left heart syndrome who may not be candidates for a stage I Norwood procedure. In the hybrid procedure, which does not require cardiopulmonary bypass, a vascular stent is placed in the patent ductus arteriosus (PDA) while bilateral pulmonary banding is performed to limit pulmonary blood flow.

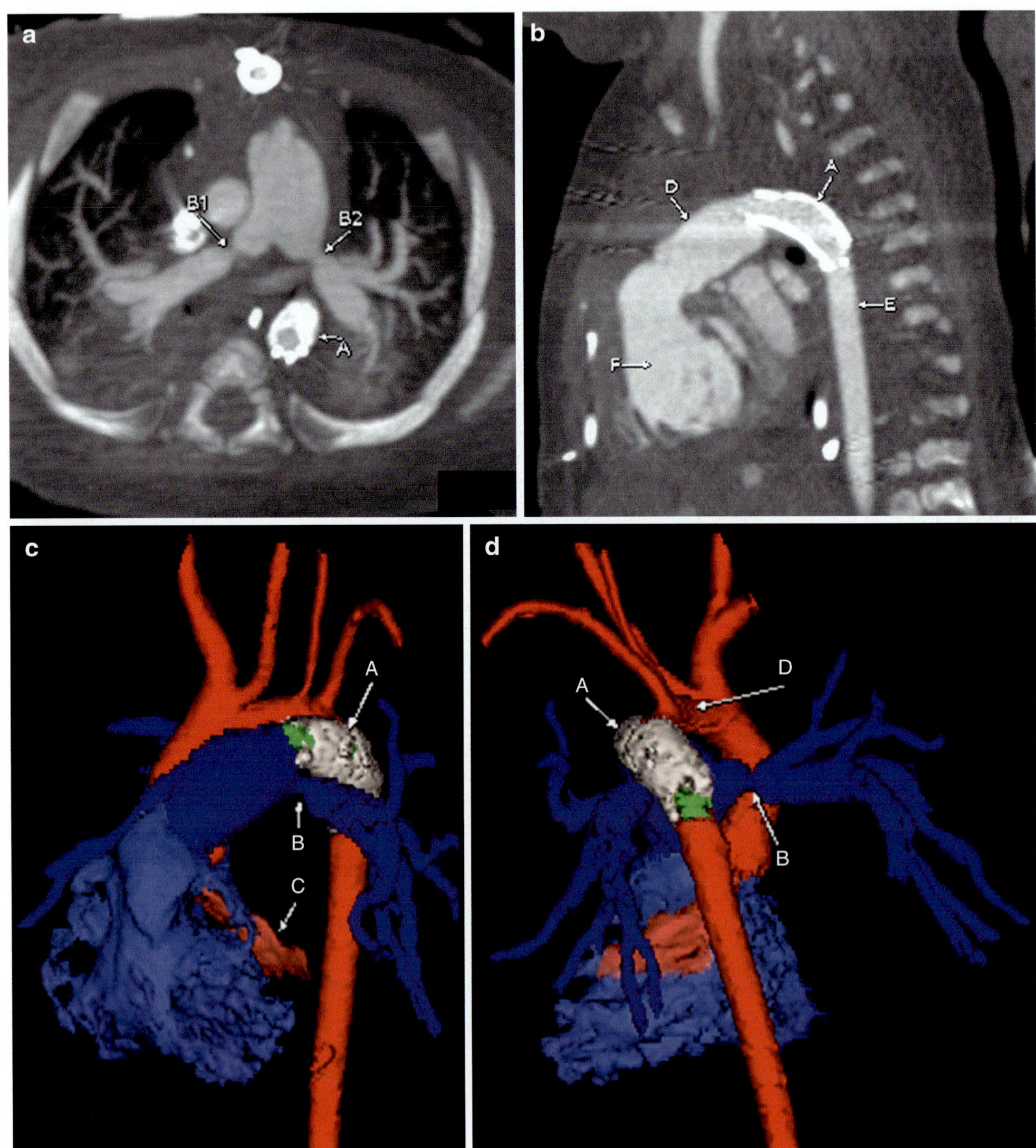

Fig. 11.5 Axial (**a**) and sagittal (**b**) CT images and lateral (**c**) and posterior (**d**) projection color-coded 3D images showing a stent (*A*, *white*) in the PDA (*green*). Notice that the PDA stent (*A*) is across the connection between the transverse aortic arch (*D*) and the descending aorta (*E*), but the holes in the stent allow retrograde flow to the transverse arch. Also note the narrow proximal right and left pulmonary arteries (*B*, *B1*, *B2*) from bilateral pulmonary artery banding. The left ventricle (*C*) is markedly hypoplastic compared with the right ventricle (*F*, *light blue*)

Norwood Procedure

The Norwood procedure is a three-part surgery performed for single-ventricle circulation, such as in patients with hypoplastic left heart syndrome. In part I (Norwood), the main pulmonary artery is disconnected from the right and left pulmonary arteries and connected to the upper portion of the aorta, creating a neoaorta. The aortic arch is widened, if necessary, with homograft tissue. A modified BT and/or Sano shunt is placed, and the atrial septum is resected. In part II (Glenn shunt), the SVC is attached to the pulmonary arteries, the modified BT shunt is taken down, and a patch is placed in the superior aspect of the right atrium. Part III (fenestrated Fontan) usually is performed at 12–24 months of age. During this stage, a graft is placed to channel blood from the IVC to the pulmonary arteries. A fenestration is created between the graft and left atrium to decompress if needed.

Norwood Part I

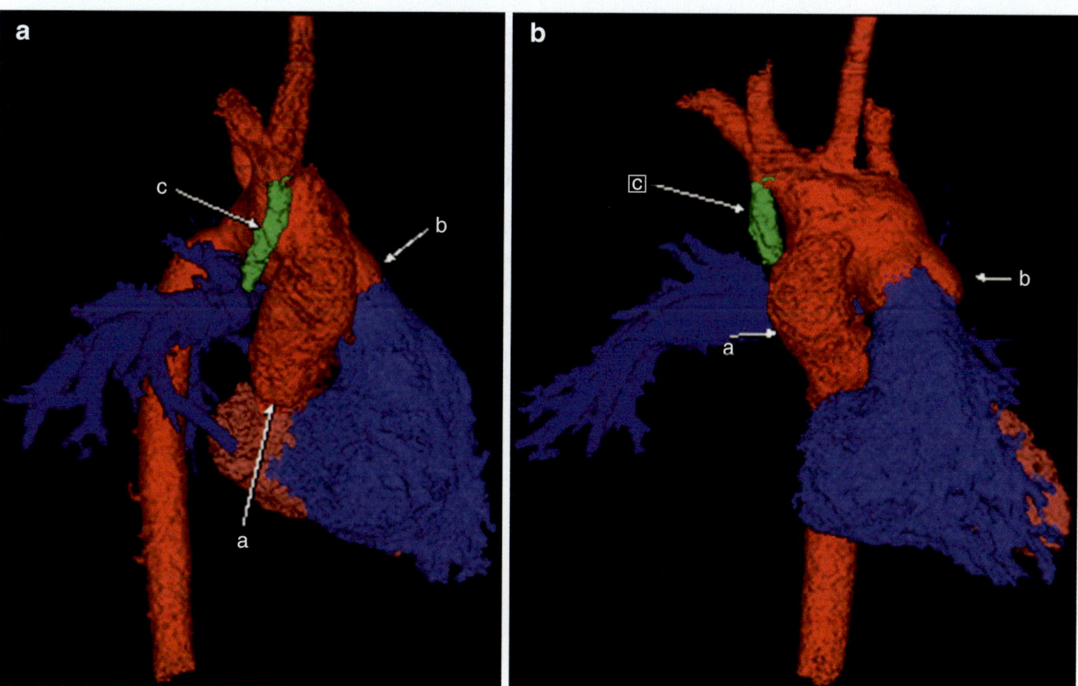

Fig. 11.6 (**a**, **b**) Color-coded 3D images showing a neoaorta (*red*) created by joining the main pulmonary artery (*b*) with the ascending aorta (*a*). A vascular conduit (*c*) connects the brachiocephalic artery to the right pulmonary artery, compatible with the modified BT shunt (*c*)

Norwood Part II

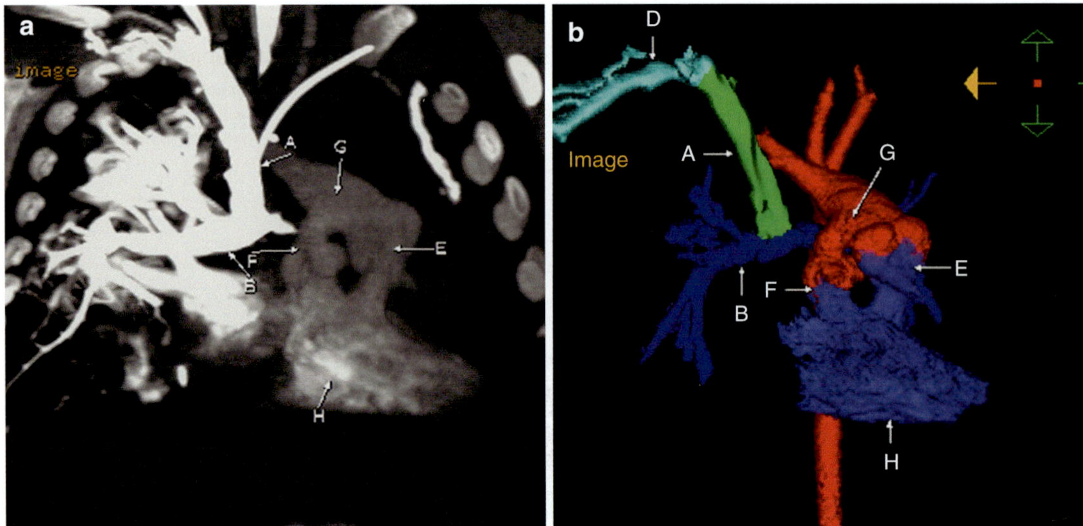

Fig. 11.7 Coronal MIP (**a**) and color-coded 3D (**b**) images from a cardiac CTA scan showing a Glenn shunt connecting the SVC (*A*) to the right pulmonary artery (*B*). Notice the neoaorta (*G*) created by joining the main pulmonary artery with the ascending aorta. Also notice that the right (*E*) and left (*F*) ventricular outflow tracts come off the right ventricle (*H*), which is the only functional ventricle

Norwood Part III

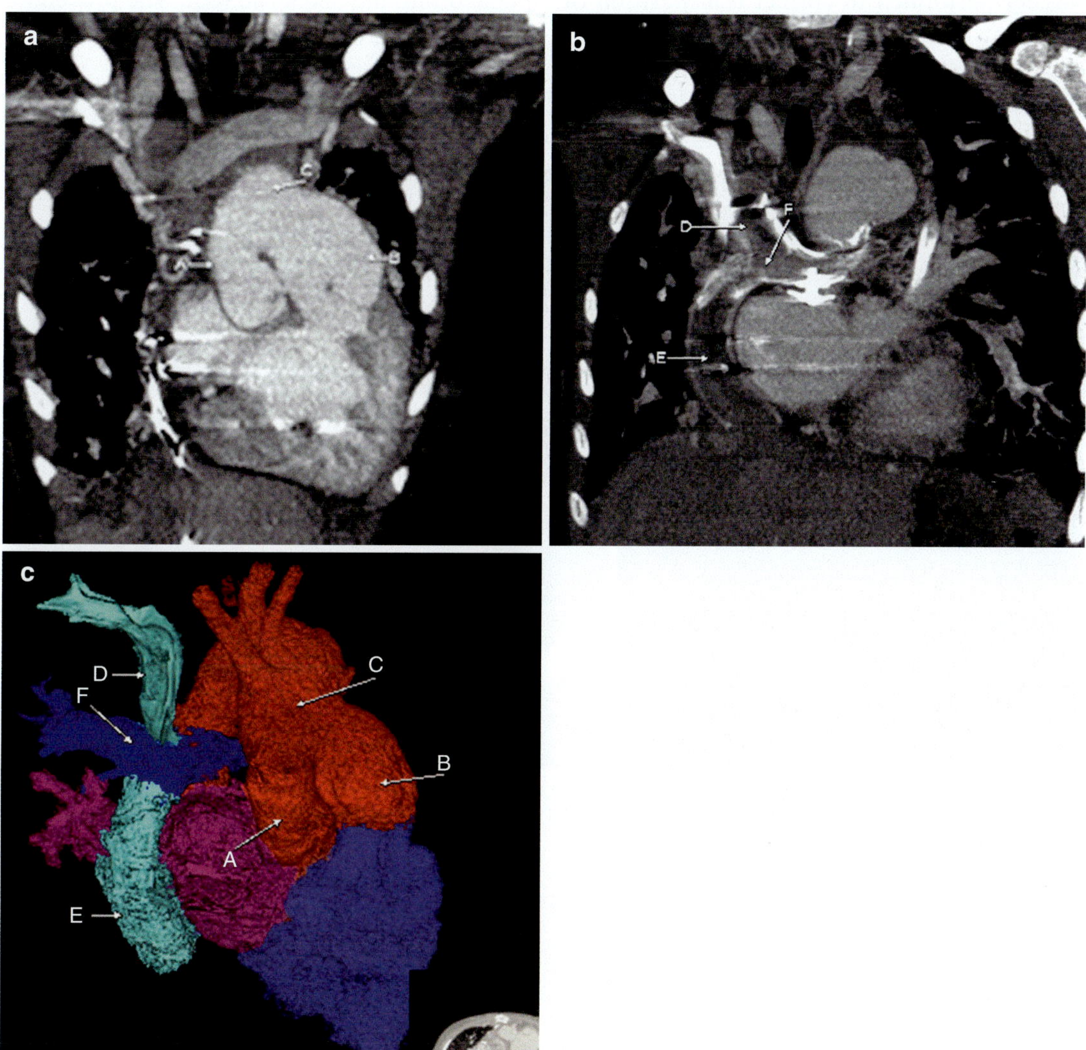

Fig. 11.8 Coronal CT (**a, b**) and color-coded 3D (**c**) images showing the result of a Norwood part III operation, with an extra-atrial Fontan shunt (*E*) channeling blood around the atrium (*pink*) to the pulmonary artery (*F*). A Glenn shunt also is present, with the SVC (*D*) shunting blood to the main pulmonary artery (*F*). Notice the neoaorta (*C*) created by joining the main pulmonary artery (*B*) with the ascending aorta (*A*)

Arterial Switch or Jatene Procedure

The arterial switch or Jatene procedure is a surgery performed to correct transposition of the great arteries. The aorta and pulmonary artery are switched, resulting in the typical "straddled" appearance of the pulmonary arteries draped around the ascending aorta. The coronary arteries are transected and reimplanted into the neoaortic root. The procedure typically is performed during the first few weeks of life.

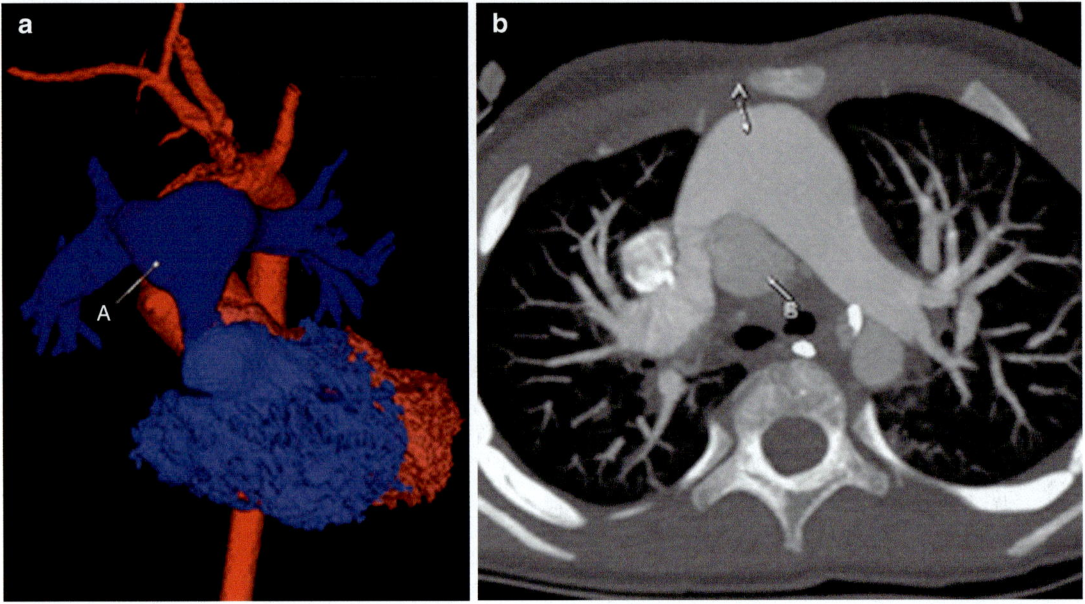

Fig. 11.9 Color-coded 3D (**a**) and axial MIP (**b**) images from a cardiac CTA scan showing the main pulmonary artery (*A*) anterior to the aorta (*B*) status post arterial switch procedure. Notice how the right and left main pulmonary arteries are draped around the ascending aorta

Fig. 11.10 Axial (**a**) and coronal (**b**) MIP images and color-coded 3D images (**c** and **d**) from a cardiac CTA scan showing the SVC (*A*) and IVC (*B*) draining into the left atrium (*C*). Deoxygenated blood then pumps from the left ventricle to the pulmonary arteries (*blue*). Oxygenated blood then returns blood to the right atrium (*F*) via the pulmonary veins (*E*). The right ventricle (*purple*) pumps blood to the aorta (*red*) in this patient with dextrotransposition of the great arteries status post Mustard procedure. Notice the typical appearance of the atrial appendage of the left atrium (*D*)

Mustard Procedure

Historically, the Mustard procedure has been performed in patients with transposition of the great arteries. It currently is not the surgery of choice for transposition repair, except in patients with L-type transposition of the great arteries, in which both the venous and arterial systems must be switched. During the Mustard procedure, the pulmonary veins are baffled to the right atrium and the SVC and IVC are baffled to the left atrium. The mustard procedure results in diverted oxygenated blood to the right ventricle, which pumps it to the body, and deoxygenated blood to the left ventricle, which pumps it to the lungs in patients with transposition.

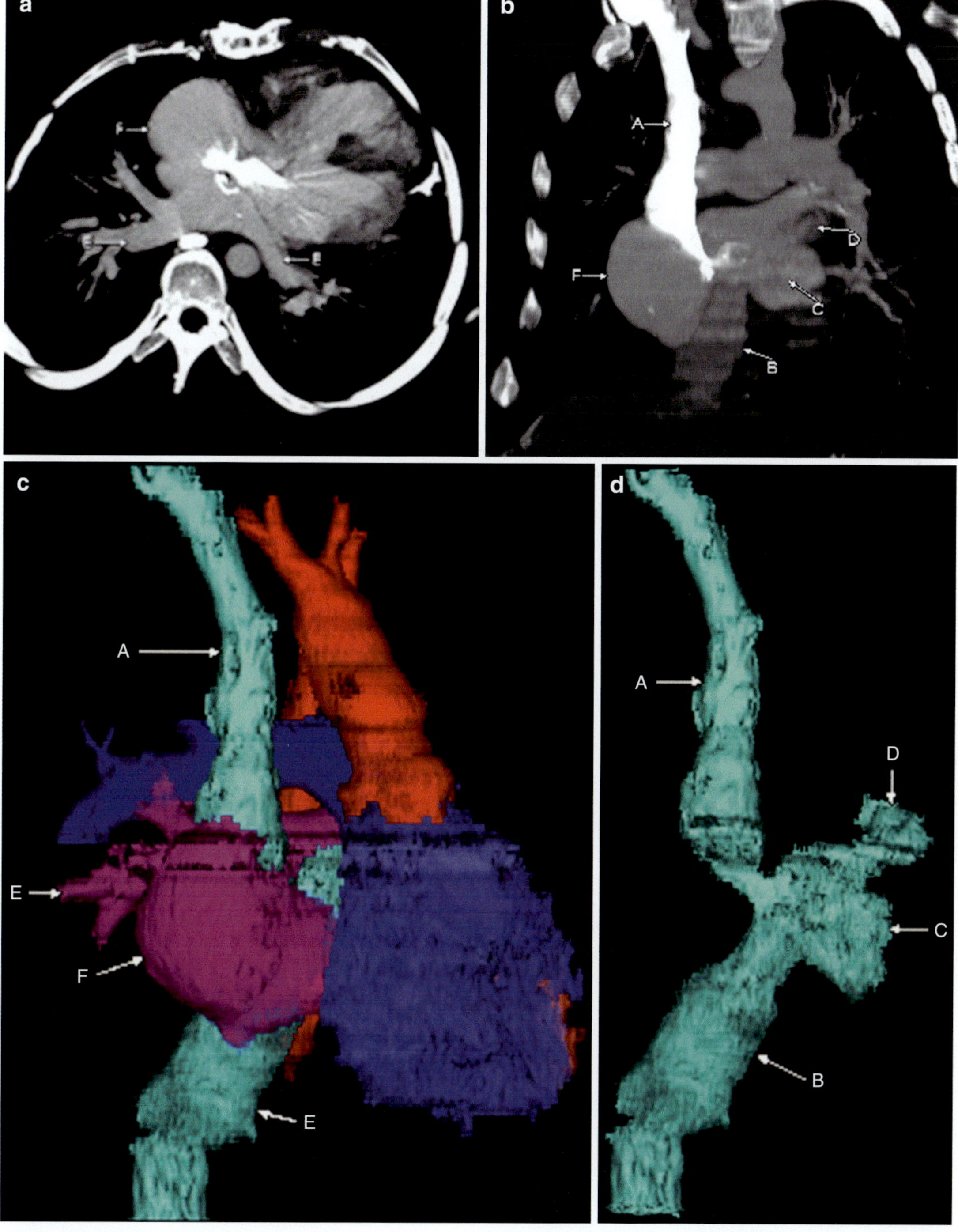

Bibliography

Bodhey NK et al. Functional analysis of the components of the right ventricle in the setting of tetralogy of Fallot. Circ Cardiovasc Imaging. 2008;1(2):141–7.

Kim YM et al. Three-dimensional computed tomography in children with compression of the central airways complicating congenital heart disease. Cardiol Young. 2002;12(1):44–50.

Krishnamurthy R. Neonatal cardiac imaging. Pediatr Radiol. 2010;40(4):518–27.

Lapierre C et al. Segmental approach to imaging of congenital heart disease. Radiographics. 2010;30(2):397–411.

Long YG et al. Role of multi-slice and three-dimensional computed tomography in delineating extracardiac vascular abnormalities in neonates. Pediatr Neonatol. 2010;51(4):227–34.

Lovato L et al. Role and effectiveness of cardiovascular magnetic resonance in the diagnosis, preoperative evaluation and follow-up of patients with congenital heart diseases. Radiol Med. 2007;112(5):660–80.

Watanabe N et al. Tracheal compression due to an elongated aortic arch in patients with congenital heart disease: evaluation using multidetector-row CT. Pediatr Radiol. 2009;39(10):1048–53.

R.R. Richardson, *Atlas of Pediatric Cardiac CTA*,
DOI 10.1007/978-1-4614-0088-2, © Springer Science+Business Media New York 2013

Index

R.R. Richardson, *Atlas of Pediatric Cardiac CTA*,
DOI 10.1007/978-1-4614-0088-2, © Springer Science+Business Media New York 2013

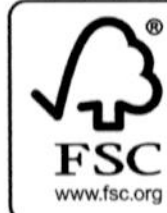

MIX
Papier aus verantwortungsvollen Quellen
Paper from responsible sources
FSC® C105338

If you have any concerns about our products,
you can contact us on
ProductSafety@springernature.com

In case Publisher is established outside the EU,
the EU authorized representative is:
Springer Nature Customer Service Center GmbH
Europaplatz 3, 69115 Heidelberg, Germany

Printed by Libri Plureos GmbH
in Hamburg, Germany